THE COMPLETE
5-INGREDIENT
DIABETIC
COOKBOOK

Simple and Easy Recipes for Busy People on Diabetic Diet

4-Week
Meal Plan

WESLEY ROBINSON

Disclaimer Notice:

Please note the information contained within this document is for educational and entertainment purposes only. All effort has been executed to present accurate, up to date, reliable, complete information. No warranties of any kind are declared or implied. Readers acknowledge that the author is not engaged in the rendering of legal, financial, medical or professional advice. The content within this book has been derived from various sources. Please consult a licensed professional before attempting any techniques outlined in this book.

By reading this document, the reader agrees that under no circumstances is the author responsible for any losses, direct or indirect, that are incurred as a result of the use of the information contained within this document, including, but not limited to, errors, omissions, or inaccuracies.

CONTENT

Part I The Basics of Diabetic Dietary

Part II 5-Ingredient Recipes

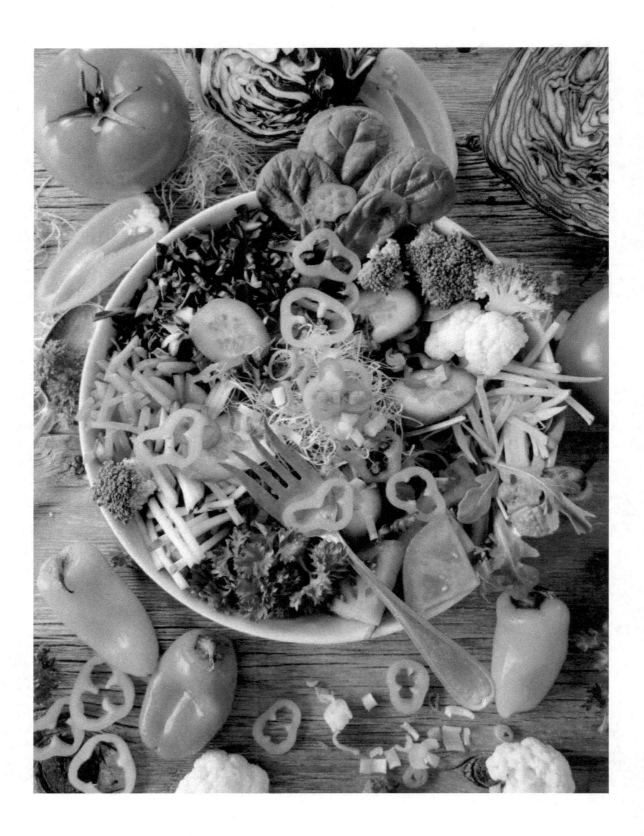

PART I

THE BASICS OF
DIABETIC DIETARY

Chapter 1: Help—I Have Diabetes!

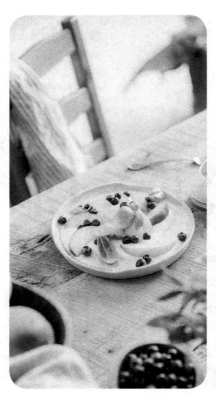

You went to the doctor because you were perhaps feeling ill, struggled to heal from minor cuts or bruises seemed to linger longer than they should. Perhaps you were always thirsty or you used the toilet more than was usual. Whatever your motivation, you got the bad news: **You're diabetic!**

My doctor, knowing that I wasn't really all that medically minded, told me the basics in a very interesting way, and it made sense, so I'd like to share it with you:

You see, our body has a funny way of turning all of our carbohydrate-rich food into sugar. So, even though I hadn't been eating bags of sugar, I had somehow ended up with way too much sugar in my bloodstream than was good for me. Now, this does not make your body a sweet place to live; instead, that sugar is like rust, and it sticks to everything in your body, messing up all your systems (heart, eyes, guts, and even your nerves).

Of course, your body is resilient, and your pancreas creates this really cool hormone called insulin, which is like a key, and it goes around your body, opening all the cells, so the sugar can go where it belongs (instead of in your bloodstream) and can actually do good things like give you energy to run or gym. Normally, that sorts out the excess sugars and your body becomes balanced again.

But sometimes, sadly, your body resists the insulin, and you have a problem … You have diabetes.

The World of Diabetes: Know Your Type

As soon as your body starts resisting the efforts of insulin, you have what is known as type 2 diabetes. Your pancreas, being a good little soldier, isn't willing to give up the fight, and it goes into overdrive, making more and more insulin, but then it runs out of juice. The insulin starts pushing more and more sugar into your cells, but this can't be sustained, and you run out of insulin. This is why people with type 2 diabetes have to regularly check their sugar (or blood glucose) levels. Luckily, we get a nifty little machine that can do this. Knowing what your sugar levels are helps you make a better decision about what to eat, when to eat, and how much to eat of any carbohydrate-containing foods.

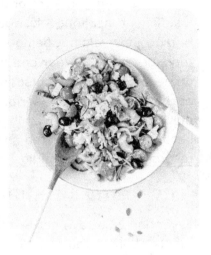

This is how you balance your sugar levels on a daily basis. However, finding that balance can be tricky, and while you can test, it doesn't help you find that personal sweet spot to keep you on track. Knowledge and informed decisions will help you get there.

Knowing the type of diabetes you have is the first step:

Prediabetes

When you tend to have more sugar or glucose levels in your blood than is considered normal, you can be said to have prediabetes. This means you are starting to become a diabetic. You may notice almost no symptoms, but the effects are cumulative, and if not addressed, you will find yourself developing type 2 diabetes.

Type 1 Diabetes

Some children have a natural tendency for their immune system to turn on their own bodies. Usually, this causes the body's own defense to destroy the insulin-producing beta cells in the pancreas. As a result, their bodies do not make insulin. In this case, insulin medication and management is required. Without enough insulin, you can suffer glycemic shock, slip into a coma, and die. While diet plays a huge role in managing all forms of diabetes, you need to combine your doctor's treatment with the 5-ingredient diabetic-diet.

Type 2 Diabetes

The more common form of diabetes among adults, type 2 diabetes results from insufficient insulin levels. You will lack energy and suffer a range of symptoms due to glucose levels not being sufficient or excessive. It's a bit like having a moody teenager living in your body: one minute you're high, the next you are arguing or sleepy, and then you suddenly have bad skin and need to pee at the strangest of times. On the more serious end of the scale, the extra glucose could lead to numbness in your extremities, and that small papercut you barely noticed could become a raging infected sore within a few days as your immune system fails to respond the way it should.

Preventing Prediabetes

Prevention is always better than cure. If you can stop yourself from developing diabetes before you actually have it, you will be saving yourself from a lifetime of being a prisoner to your body. It isn't even all that difficult.

Research has proven that if you are prediabetic, you can decrease the chances of the onset of type 2 diabetes by losing 7% of your body mass and following a moderate exercise routine. Something as simple as a daily walk around your neighborhood could save your life.

Should you already have type 2 diabetes, this is not a death sentence. You are not "deadman walking," and by maintaining a healthy weight, engaging in regular exercise, and eating wisely, you can improve your body's acceptance of insulin, thereby decreasing the sugar levels in your blood. You can lock the moody-diabetes-teenager away and live a healthy and fulfilling life.

Diabetes Treatment Options

Treating diabetes is not about getting rid of some boogie in your life. Instead, it is about management. Once diagnosed as diabetic, most people don't magically unbecome diabetic. This means you can't hide in your closet and refuse to deal with the reality and impact of diabetes on your health.

You need to use medical treatment, dietary treatment, and a combination of physical activity and balanced mental health to keep yourself in good health.

Medical Treatment

When treating and managing your diabetes, you need to know your blood sugar levels. If you don't know your "sweet spot," you won't be able to regulate your intake of carbohydrates or sucrose and production of insulin. For type 1 diabetes, this becomes crucial as you may need to take insulin injections to help regulate your blood sugar.

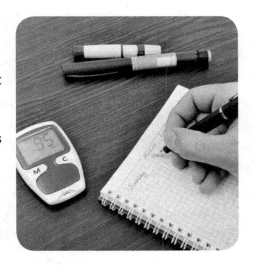

Testing your blood sugar levels isn't like randomly checking your bank balance at the ATM. You need to be organized—your life may depend on it.

When you are a diagnosed as a diabetic, you need to be prepared and diligent in your testing:

- Always keep your testing equipment with you.

- Use new testing strips and keep them away from heat and sunlight.

- Make testing part of your life and test at the same times each day.

- Schedule maintenance and calibration of your testing machine regularly.

- Keep track of your results in a notebook or app on your phone.

- Manage your testing site effectively and safely.

Knowing what your sugar levels are helps you plan your diet and enables you to manage your diabetes with careful nutrition planning.

Dietary Treatment

Medical Nutrition Therapy (MNT) is when your healthcare practitioner advises you about which foods to avoid, which to bulk on, and times and quantities of your meals. This helps your body work in sync with your unique diabetes diagnosis. No two diabetics are identical, and while you can maybe sneak a candy bar once in a while, your neighbor may have fits if they have even one sniff of chocolate.

In numerous tests and research studies, the DASH diet, the Mediterranean diet, and vegetarian or plant-based foods have been found to be the most beneficial to those managing their diabetes. After all, you are what you eat.

A structured meal plan can really help you get those blood sugar numbers under control. By following a specially crafted MNT, you can cut down on the blood glucose levels in your body, reducing your blood sugar levels, and maintaining optimal health. This puts you in control of your diabetes with every spoonful you eat.

Physical Activity and Mental Health

Get up and move. Not only will this help you produce endorphins that will help you feel better, it will also reduce your blood glucose levels. Even if you don't necessarily lose weight with your physical activities, it is still a win for anyone living with diabetes.

Try to get at least two and a half hours of physical activity throughout a week. Be careful to spread that feel-good movement over a couple of days. Never do more than two consecutive days of exercise. Not only will this help prevent injuries, but it will also help you form healthy physical activity habits.

Living with diabetes can be overwhelming, and you need to cultivate a strong mental approach. Type 2 diabetes is particularly rough on your emotions, and you may suffer from mood swings and feel stressed. Engage in self-care, and you will be able to remain mentally and emotionally fit and on top of your game.

If you are going to let sugar become your boss, then your health will suffer. Diabetes management is important to preserve your health and well-being. Stay positive and live responsibly. There is no need to become overwhelmed or depressed (though you may feel like this at times). When in doubt, reach out. There are amazing online support groups, such as diabetesteam.com or thediabetessupportgroup.org. And in many urban centers, there are also diabetes clinics where you can get access to resources and helpful advice from medical professionals.

Diabetes is absolutely treatable, and by following a controlled diet, working with your healthcare practitioners, and maintaining a healthy weight and exercise program (and, if necessary, taking medication), you can beat diabetes.

Chapter 2: Nutrition and Diabetes

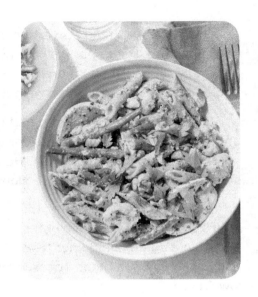

Designing your diet to support and manage your diabetes is often a daunting challenge. What can you eat? Should youMacronutrients avoid all sugar or carbohydrates? How do you make sure to still get enough nutrients to ensure good health?

These are all valid questions, and while you may be able to consult a dietician, it is still helpful to know the basics and be able to stir your own pot (so to speak). A balanced diet is essential to manage diabetes and avoid causing other health problems. While cutting carbs and calories may help you lose weight and lower your blood glucose levels, this could cause you to become anemic, suffer digestive disorders, and even plunge you further into depression with type 2 diabetes.

The idea is to live better and healthier, not starve yourself. You do not have to buy expensive commercialized "meals for diabetics," and it is up to you to find what works on your budget, for your tastes, and according to your unique dietary needs.

Macronutrients

These basic building blocks are what you will structure your diet around as they provide the fuel your body requires to function:

Carbohydrates

Sources: Quinoa, brown rice, barley, and fresh vegetables and fruits.

You don't have to cut out all carbs or starches, even though these can become converted to glucose in your bloodstream. For starters, carbs are not all equal. Carbs are found in simple and complex form, and the simple carbs found in dairy and vegetables are essential building blocks that are good for you. Your body also gets most of its energy supply from carbs. While fruits are also rich in carbs, they contain larger amounts of sucrose or sugars, which are not friends with your blood glucose levels.

Overall, you should strive to consume foods with complex carbs as they are packed with nutrients, and since they digest slower, they don't flood your system with a flash of sugars. Being more filling, they also make you eat less, suppress cravings, and as a result, you will lose weight. Great news for those with type 2 diabetes.

Fiber-rich sources of grain and natural starches are great sources of whole grain and complex carbs. They make for great fillers in your diet. Adults should consume 45-60 grams of carbs per meal. Hence, if you want to feel full and not like you're starving, you need to consume slow-releasing carbs.

By knowing the Glycemic Index (GI) of the foods in your diet, you can plan your meals so you can have enough slow release sources of carbs to keep you fuller and maintain a sustainable energy level. The lower the number of your GI, the less your body sees a rise in blood sugar levels. This is why we see so many foods labeled as low GI foods.

Glycemic Load (GL) is another consideration when planning your meals. This is a scale that helps you to know how quickly you are likely to increase your blood sugar levels after eating one gram of carb rich food.

As a golden rule with carbs, you should limit simple carbs, avoid added sugars, and you should aim to consume whole (or complex) carbs or fiber-rich carbs.

Protein

Sources: Fish, lean cut meats, dairy products, eggs, and red meats (try to limit these).

Including protein in your diet is also a way to gain value from another energy source. It's like having a car that runs on fuel and on electricity. As an added benefit, eating protein and carbs together is a great way to ensure your sugar levels remain more stable as protein digests slower than carbs, which is probably why you feel so full after a great Christmas lunch.

Protein is found from two sources, namely plant-based and animal-based proteins. Plant proteins contain extra fiber, which will help regulate your digestive system, and these also go down much easier on your kidneys. While science seems to indicate that eating plant-based proteins is most beneficial for those who are type 2 diabetics, you can still enjoy all the benefits by simply tailoring your diet to include more plant-based protein, and you don't have to become vegan or vegetarian at all.

Fat

Sources: **Fatty fish like salmon and anchovies, seeds like chia seeds, olive oil, nuts, avocado, leafy green vegetables, and olives.**

We all know the concept of burning fat. It's why you slave away at the gym, trying to burn fat off your bum, isn't it? Nope. Body fat is simply stored up energy. However, the fats you should be eating are called unsaturated fats. As a rule of thumb, they are in a liquid state at room temperature.

Polyunsaturated fats such as the oils or fatty acids in fish are considered essential fats, and these are really important to your diet as your body can't produce them. Omega-3 fatty acids are an example of these, and you should also consume monounsaturated fats like those found in avocados.

You should avoid trans fats (hydrogenated fats) as much as possible. This is when fat has been altered by manufacturers to include an extra hydrogen molecule. These fats are dangerous to your health as they are unnatural and raise cholesterol.

Other Essential Nutrients to Add or Avoid

Vitamin D

Sources: **Swordfish, salmon, tuna, sardines, eggs, and Shiitake mushrooms.**

A diet deficient in vitamin D is associated with a decrease in insulin production. For those living with type 2 diabetes, this is bad news. Make sure that you add sources of vitamin D rich food to your diet.

Magnesium

Sources: **Leafy green vegetables, seeds, nuts, avocados, and legumes.**

This mineral is essential for a whole range of processes in your body. Be sure to include substantial amounts of sources rich in magnesium in your diet to successfully manage your blood pressure, regulate cell health, produce essential neurotransmitters, and to decrease the risk of developing type 2 diabetes.

> ## Sodium
>
> **Sources:** **Processed foods such as take-aways, commercial sauces, and packaged foods like potato crisps, dried meats, and processed juices.**
>
> Sodium may be a great preservative and flavorant, and it certainly adds the yum to many processed foods, but it is VERY unhealthy for you. Since it increases the risk of developing heart disease, high blood pressure, and having a stroke, it is also a big no-no for you if you are managing diabetes. I advise cutting it out of your diet as much as possible—this isn't normal table salt though, which isn't sodium at all. So, check your labels to see what the sodium content of a product is before you add it to your shopping cart and to your body.

Preparing for Your Diabetes Dietary Choices

Living with diabetes is not a death sentence, and you can easily manage your health and enjoy your meals with a little knowledge and some careful preparation. Be sure to focus on eating whole foods, which aren't processed as these contain more "good" fats, fewer simple carbs, and less sodium. Most vegetables and lean meats are considered whole foods, and they contain all the essential nutrients you need, as well as all the amino acids your health requires. As a bonus, these are usually slow to digest, leaving you feeling fuller for longer—so you'll have less cravings and be able to fit into that summer bikini much easier.

Get informed. You need to know what you are putting in your body. Once you know what moves past your teeth, you will be in control, and you can then make the necessary adjustments to maintain healthy insulin and blood glucose levels. Diabetes can be managed by careful dietary choices. The good news is: once you get used to eating this way, it gets easier and so much more fun too (just wait till you see my yummy recipes).

When you live with diabetes, you should know how many carbs your body is absorbing with each meal. This is known as net carbs. With whole foods, simply subtract the fiber amount, which leaves you with the carbs total. As a diabetic, you should count the grams of your food, matching every 15 grams (or one carb serving) to your insulin levels.

You should also stay informed of the latest developments and get support for your diabetes management. The American Diabetes Association offers online resources to advocate responsible meal design, while you can also use a handy app such as Carb Manager from the Play store, which lets you track carbs, net carbs, and manage what you eat and when you eat.

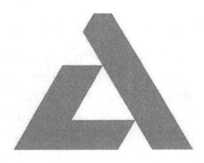

Reading a food label is an important skill for a healthy diet. When you read a label, you should make sure to get the following information:

1. Serving size

2. Calories per serving

3. The contribution by the "badies" to the carb count. So, look at the amount of fat (especially trans fats), sodium, cholesterol, preservatives, etc. in that carb count. You should avoid foods that have high volumes of these as they are not healthy.

4. Check the carbohydrate, fiber, and protein content as well as the content of other useful nutrients like vitamins, minerals, and healthy fats.

5. Study the overall percentages of each component and the daily value/daily recommendation (DV/DR) of each. If you are already getting 100% of the daily recommended value of carbs in one serving of pasta, for instance, then you need to reconsider this food as your daily dietary allowance will become unbalanced.

6. Also look at the list of ingredients to avoid colorants, flavorants, and preservatives that are equally bad for your health.

This may seem a bit like the classic Western movie: The Good, The Bad, and The Ugly, but you will get used to seeing a label and knowing what is good, what is bad, and what is down-right ugly.

Food List and Portions

When dealing with carbs, we consider 15 grams to be a single carb serving. This works out well as it allows you a single slice of bread for a full carb serving. Knowing what the quantities are for different foods to obtain the same amount of carbs is essential to planning a nutritious and balanced meal. You can also use an app such as MyPlate to track and check the calorie content of each meal you prepare. Here's a couple of basic food lists to get you started, and each single carb serving is equal to 15 grams of carbs for each of the food categories:

Starch

- ► ½ cup each of cooked oatmeal, green peas, sweet potato, corn, cooked beans, cooked lentils, or plantain
- ► ⅓ cup each of brown rice or whole-wheat pasta (cooked), quinoa (cooked)
- ► 1 cup winter squash
- ► 1 slice of whole-wheat bread or ½ a whole-wheat English muffin
- ► ¾ cup of cold non-sugary cereal
- ► ½ potato (medium size)
- ► 1 corn cob or tortilla (flour based)

Fruits

- ► ½ each of a grapefruit or a banana
- ► 1 small fruit each, like a pear, an apple, an orange, a peach, or a nectarine
- ► 2-3 small guavas or plums, or dried prunes
- ► 12 grapes
- ► ¾ cup of blueberries or fresh pineapple
- ► ⅔ cup of cherries (pitted)

Dairy Products Such as Milk and Yoghurt

- ► 6 ounces each of plain yoghurt or plain Greek yoghurt (a higher protein source)
- ► 8 ounces of full-fat organic milk or unsweetened soy milk (as it's denser, it will not raise your blood sugar too quickly)

Non-Starchy Veggies

As a quick rule, these are not as carbohydrate rich as other vegetables, so each serving size only contains 5 grams of carbs. This means you can have three times the guided amount to make up a single carb serving. A serving size (5 grams of carbs) is usually ½ cup cooked veggies or 1 cup raw veggies. You can consider these: green beans, Brussels sprouts, broccoli, mushrooms, zucchini, salads, and cabbage.

Snacks

- ▶ ¾ ounce each crackers or pretzels
- ▶ 3 cups popcorn (air-popped without oil or butter or low-fat microwave variety)
- ▶ 10-12 potato crisps

It is probably best to check the labels of each of the snacks you consider eating for a more accurate guide with snacks.

Watch What You Eat

You should be mindful of the impact of your meals on your health, your blood sugar levels, and your ability to live a productive life. One sure way I control my weight and my health is to practice portion control.

Portion Size

When working out your portion size, you need to be aware of what is actually in every spoonful that passes your lips. This may sound dreadful, but it isn't.

As a guide, when maintaining your current body weight:

- You should eat 10 calories per pound of your own weight daily if you are overweight and lead a lifestyle that is mostly sedentary.

- If you are a little overweight but exercise regularly, then you should consume 13 calories per pound of your own body weight each day.

- With physically active and weight-controlled people, you can eat upwards of 15 calories per pound of your own body weight per day.

Alcohol

If you are fond of your wine or other forms of alcohol, you need to take cognizance of the fact that alcohol is often produced through fermentation that includes the adding of sugars. Beer and sweet variety wines contain added sugars and are high in carbs, which can make your blood sugar spike instantly. However, alcohol can also cause your blood sugar to plummet, causing hypoglycemia or low blood sugar levels. Keep this in mind when indulging in your favorite beverage.

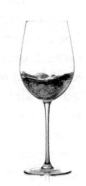

Sugar Substitutes

When you are trying to lose weight or have been diagnosed with diabetes, you'll quickly throw out those spoonfuls of sugar in your tea or coffee. Alternative sweeteners such as Stevia, Tagatose, and Sucralose are popular and available in a variety of forms on the market. Sweeten your tea or coffee with one or two tablets or a sachet and watch pounds drop while you maintain a steady blood sugar level.

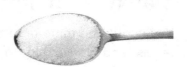

Chapter 3: Starting Your Diabetic Diet Journey

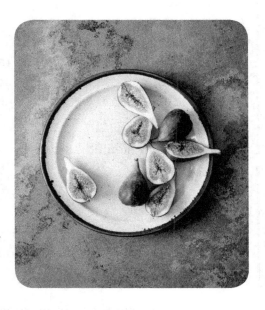

Armed with knowledge, you are now ready to start anew. If you're like me, you are probably standing in your kitchen, looking at all the nice things you can't eat anymore and wondering where to start. Don't despair! Let's start with where you serve from—your plate.

The Plate Method

This is a very easy way to control what you eat. Firstly, start with a 9-inch plate. You should measure it to be sure about the size. Remember, the bigger your plate, the more you'll dish up, and the more you'll put into your body. So, 9 inches, no more.

The plate method is a popular theory that helps with weight loss, weight management, and calorie control. Each meal is served according to the following size guides:

- ½ plate of non-starchy vegetables (any veggie with fewer than 5 grams of carbs per serving)

- ¼ plate healthy protein (animal or plant-based is fine)

- ¼ high fiber carbs (no more than 15 grams for women or 30 grams for men)

You can also add some healthy fats but no more than 5-6 spoonfuls as part of a salad dressing, nuts or seeds, or in the meal prep for your food. Additionally, you may also notice that your plate is usually not full. This may sound crazy. But you should fill your plate, especially the ½ plate of non-starchy veggies. Most of us don't eat enough veggies and we don't consume nearly enough fiber. Don't forget to add your small cup of dairy such as yogurt or fruit to your daily intake too.

Create the Right Kitchen

Now that your plate is sorted, it's time to get your kitchen diabetic-friendly and wrapped in awesomeness. While you may want to rush out and buy the latest beautiful appliances, fryers, and inspirational kitchen tools, you don't have to. Chances are that you'll end up not using half of these if you rush. So, rather start with the basics:

In Your Pantry

While some of the diabetic cooking recipes may be a little different in taste than your usual cooking, you can literally swallow anything if you spice it well, and as your tastebuds change, you will start to enjoy these recipes immensely. Stock up your pantry with the following to boost and flavor your recipes:

► almonds and almond butter

► anchovy paste

► pearl barley

► dried basil, bay leaves, oregano, onion powder and flakes, paprika, pepper, sage, salt, thyme, pumpkin seeds, and cherries

► gluten-free bread crumbs

► cashews, peanuts, and other omega rich nuts

► chia and hemp seeds

► chili powder, cinnamon, cloves, coriander, curry powder, ginger, fennel and flaxseed (ground)

► coconut flakes and cocoa powder (unsweetened)

► cornstarch, baking powder, and whole-wheat flour

► canola, olive, coconut, and sesame oils

► vinegars (apple cider, balsamic, red wine, rice wine and apple cider)

► pure vanilla extract

In Your Fridge

Make sure your fridge is clean and well stocked to inspire success in your health and meal planning. Always keep these basics on hand:

▶ eggs

▶ fresh veggies (pre-washed and chopped cuts down on meal prep time)

▶ fresh protein sources such as fish and poultry (store these separately to avoid spreading contaminants)

▶ hummus or another favorite dip

▶ milk alternatives such as almond or cashew milk

▶ plain yogurt

▶ plant proteins like pre-cooked tofu, lentils, and other soy products

▶ Washed green veggies such as salads, spinach, and other leafy greens

In Your Freezer

Many of us live in the frozen foods aisle. There is nothing more convenient than frozen meals to pop in the microwave and enjoy, but this can be a source of strategic and healthy food too. By pre-cooking extra food, you can easily freeze portions and have healthy food available on demand. Make sure to stock up on these:

▶ Salmon, cod, and other seafoods

▶ Frozen lean meats such as chicken breasts, lean beef, and ground turkey

▶ Frozen berries and mixed fruits

▶ Frozen vegetables

▶ Frozen left-overs as additions to future meals

Utensils and Cooking Equipment

Some essentials to have:

▶ A food processor/blender

▶ A toaster

▶ Baking sheets, glass baking dishes, and muffin tins

▶ Graters and ice-cube trays to grate and store (freeze) leftover herbs

▶ Good quality knives (chopping and paring)

▶ One plastic (for meats) and one wooden (for veggies and cooked foods) chopping boards each

▶ Digital thermometer, measuring cups, quality sealing containers to store leftovers in.

> **You may be inspired to buy some "nice-to-haves," and you can consider these:**
>
> - A slow cooker
> - A pressure cooker (instant pot)
> - Purée maker (immersion blender)
> - Air fryer oven
>
> Now that your kitchen is set up, you can indulge in guilt-free, healthy cooking and share with the world ... but what about your friends who aren't diabetic or the coming holidays? What then? You can face special occasions with a smile.

Special Occasions

Whenever you follow a special diet, whether for health, for weight loss, or for gaining weight, going to events away from home is often tricky. When you are not the one making the food, you may have little control over what is served to you. However, you can survive these events and not be a party pooper.

Here are some helpful tips to manage your diabetes friendly diet while socializing:

- Eat something before you go out. This helps manage your ability to over-eat.

- At restaurants, order food prepared to your needs (low oil, replacing potatoes with extra veggies, or ordering baked potatoes instead of fries).

- If you are attending a social event at a friend's place, make sure to take a healthy plate as a contribution or ask them to help you with your dietary goals.

- Avoid buffets where the temptation of second servings can be overwhelming.

- Plan with a friend to take a walk after dinner, and you will find yourself planning to not overeat to keep this appointment.

- Partake in alcohol moderately and stick to dry wines.

- Where restaurants serve large portions, share with a friend, or share dessert to still satisfy your sweet craving but avoid a carb and sugar overload.

- Eat slowly as this will encourage you to eat less.

- Avoid socializing with people who don't support your health choices. Some people simply don't want to understand your dietary needs, and hanging out with them usually ends up in binge eating and sugar highs.

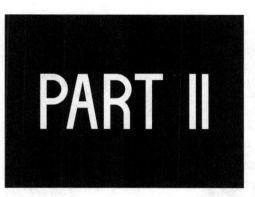

PART II

5-INGREDIENT RECIPES

You may ask why you should use five ingredients to prepare your diabetic meal plan. Simply put—it's easy. Focusing on less ingredients will ensure that you can easily balance your carbs, know your intake of carbs, and you will find flavors are fuller and more enhanced by the spices and prep you put in.

With fewer ingredients, it is easier to ensure you get a full spectrum of veggies, proteins, and healthy carbs. Additionally, you will find it much easier to prep these meals, shopping will become simpler, and you will feel an intense health benefit from the first bite.

Feeling inspired to manage your diabetic health better? Grab your spoon, and let's start cooking!

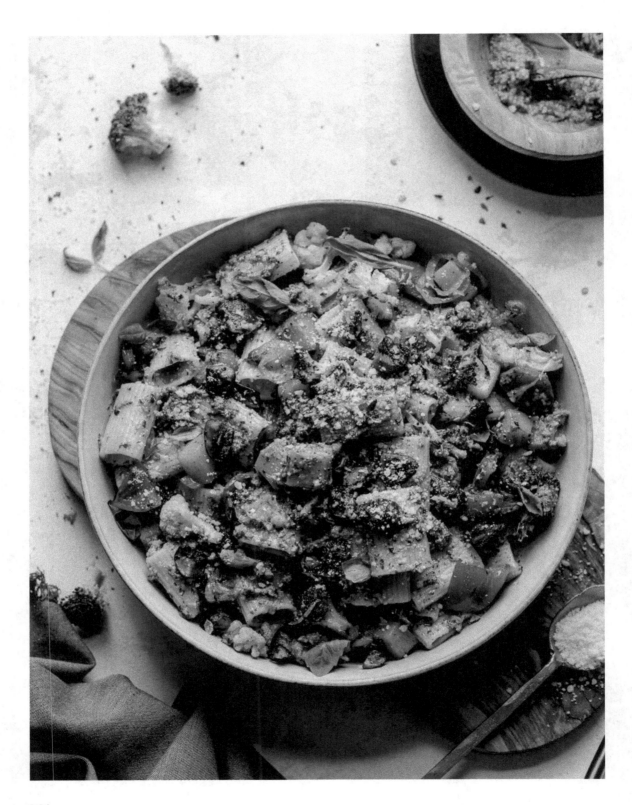

CHAPTER 4

BREAKFAST

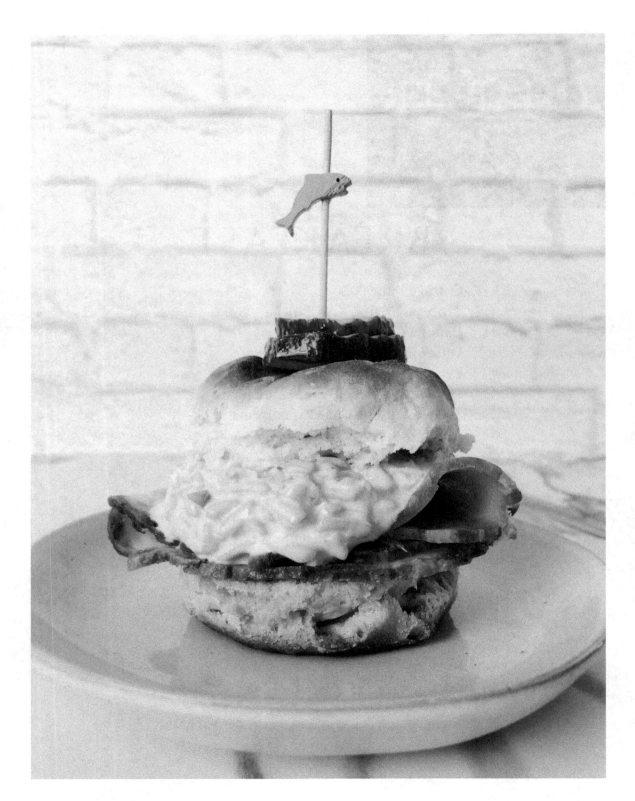

Cottage Pancakes

Prep time: 10 minutes | Cook time: 20 minutes | Serves 4

- 2 cups low-fat cottage cheese
- 4 egg whites
- 2 eggs

- 1 tablespoon pure vanilla extract
- 1½ cups almond flour

From the Cupboard:
- Nonstick cooking spray

1. Place the cottage cheese, egg whites, eggs, and vanilla in a blender and pulse to combine.
2. Add the almond flour to the blender and blend until smooth.
3. Place a large nonstick skillet over medium heat and lightly coat it with cooking spray.
4. Spoon ¼ cup of batter per pancake, 4 at a time, into the skillet. Cook the pancakes until the bottoms are firm and golden, about 4 minutes.
5. Flip the pancakes over and cook the other side until they are cooked through, about 3 minutes.
6. Remove the pancakes to a plate and repeat with the remaining batter.
7. Serve with fresh fruit.

Per Serving

calories: 345 | fat: 22.1g | protein: 29.1g | carbs: 11.1g | fiber: 4.1g | sugar: 5.1g
sodium: 560mg

Tropical Yogurt Kiwi Bowl

Prep time: 5 minutes | Cook time: 0 minutes | Serves 2

- 1½ cups plain low-fat Greek yogurt
- 2 kiwis, peeled and sliced
- 2 tablespoons shredded unsweetened

- coconut flakes
- 2 tablespoons halved walnuts
- 1 tablespoon chia seeds

1. Divide the yogurt between two small bowls.
2. Top each serving of yogurt with half of the kiwi slices, coconut flakes, walnuts, and chia seeds.

Per Serving

calories: 261 | fat: 9.1g | protein: 21.1g | carbs: 23.1g | fiber: 6.1g | sugar: 14.1g
sodium: 84mg

Banana Crêpe Cakes

- 4 ounces (113 g) reduced-fat plain cream cheese, softened
- 2 medium bananas

From the Cupboard:

- Avocado oil cooking spray

- 4 large eggs
- ½ teaspoon vanilla extract

- ⅛ teaspoon salt

1. Heat a large skillet over low heat. Coat the cooking surface with cooking spray, and allow the pan to heat for another 2 to 3 minutes.
2. Meanwhile, in a medium bowl, mash the cream cheese and bananas together with a fork until combined. The bananas can be a little chunky.
3. Add the eggs, vanilla, and salt, and mix well.
4. For each cake, drop 2 tablespoons of the batter onto the warmed skillet and use the bottom of a large spoon or ladle to spread it thin. Let it cook for 7 to 9 minutes.
5. Flip the cake over and cook briefly, about 1 minute.

Per Serving

calories: 176 | fat: 9.1g | protein: 9.1g | carbs: 15.1g | fiber: 2.1g | sugar: 8.1g
sodium: 214mg

Quick Breakfast Yogurt Sundae

- ¾ cup plain Greek yogurt
- ¼ cup mixed berries (blueberries, strawberries, blackberries)
- 2 tablespoons cashew, walnut, or

almond pieces
- 1 tablespoon ground flaxseed
- 2 fresh mint leaves, shredded

1. Pour the yogurt into a tall parfait glass and scatter the top with the berries, cashew pieces, and flaxseed.
2. Sprinkle the mint leaves on top for garnish and serve chilled.

Per Serving

calories: 238 | fat: 11.2g | protein: 20.9g | carbs: 15.8g | fiber: 4.1g | sugar: 8.9g
sodium: 63mg

Cranberry Grits

Prep time: 10 minutes | Cook time: 15 minutes | Serves 5

- ¾ cup stone-ground grits or polenta (not instant)
- ½ cup unsweetened dried cranberries
- 1 tablespoon half-and-half
- ¼ cup sliced almonds, toasted
- From the Cupboard:
- Pinch kosher salt
- 1 tablespoon unsalted butter or ghee (optional)

1. In the electric pressure cooker, stir together the grits, cranberries, salt, and 3 cups of water.
2. Close and lock the lid. Set the valve to sealing.
3. Cook on high pressure for 10 minutes.
4. When the cooking is complete, hit Cancel and quick release the pressure.
5. Once the pin drops, unlock and remove the lid.
6. Add the butter (if using) and half-and-half. Stir until the mixture is creamy, adding more half-and-half if necessary.
7. Spoon into serving bowls and sprinkle with almonds.

Per Serving

calories: 219 | fat: 10.2g | protein: 4.9g | carbs: 32.1g | fiber: 4.1g | sugar: 6.9g
sodium: 30mg

Ham and Cheese Breakfast Biscuits

Prep time: 5 minutes | Cook time: 15 minutes | Serves 4

- 1 cup ham, diced
- 2 eggs
- ¾ cup Mozzarella cheese, grated
- ½ cup low fat Cheddar cheese, grated
- ½ cup reduced fat grated Parmesan, grated

1. Heat oven to 375ºF (190ºC). Line a baking sheet with parchment paper.
2. In a large bowl, combine the cheeses and eggs until fully combined. Stir in the ham.
3. Divide the mixture evenly into 8 parts and form into round tolls. Bake for 15 to 20 minutes or until cheese is completely melted and the rolls are nicely browned.

Per Serving

calories: 193 | fat: 13.1g | protein: 16.1g | carbs: 2.2g | fiber: 0g | sugar: 0g
sodium: 1192mg

Simple Cottage Cheese Pancakes

Prep time: 5 minutes | Cook time: 10 minutes | Serves 2

Batter:

- ½ cup low-fat cottage cheese
- ¼ cup oats
- ⅓ cup egg whites (about 2 egg whites)
- 1 tablespoon stevia
- 1 teaspoon vanilla extract

From the Cupboard:

- Olive oil cooking spray

1. Add the cottage cheese, oats, egg whites, stevia and vanilla extract to a food processor. Pulse into a smooth and thick batter.
2. Coat a large skillet with cooking spray and place it over medium heat.
3. Slowly pour half of the batter into the pan, tilting the pan to spread it evenly. Cook for about 2 to 3 minutes until the pancake turns golden brown around the edges. Gently flip the pancake with a spatula and cook for 1 to 2 minutes more.
4. Transfer the pancake to a plate and repeat with the remaining batter.
5. Serve warm.

Per Serving

calories: 188 | fat: 1.6g | protein: 24.6g | carbs: 18.9g | fiber: 1.9g | sugar: 2g sodium: 258mg

Almond Berry Smoothie

Prep time: 5 minutes | Cook time: 0 minutes | Serves 4

- 2 cups frozen berries of choice
- 1 cup plain low-fat Greek yogurt
- 1 cup unsweetened vanilla almond milk
- ½ cup natural almond butter

1. In a blender, add the berries, almond milk, yogurt, and almond butter. Process until fully mixed and creamy. Pour into four smoothie glasses.
2. Serve chilled or at room temperature.

Per Serving

calories: 279 | fat: 18.2g | protein: 13.4g | carbs: 19.1g | fiber: 6.1g | sugar: 11.1g sodium: 138mg

Feta Brussels Sprouts and Scrambled Eggs

Prep time: 5 minutes | Cook time: 15 minutes | Serves 4

- 4 slices low-sodium turkey bacon
- 20 Brussels sprouts, halved lengthwise
- 8 large eggs, whisked
- ¼ cup crumbled feta cheese, for garnish
- From the Cupboard:
- Avocado oil cooking spray

1. Heat a large skillet over medium heat until hot. Coat the skillet with cooking spray.
2. Fry the bacon slices for about 8 minutes until evenly crisp, flipping occasionally.
3. With a slotted spoon, transfer the bacon to a paper towel-lined plate to drain and cool. Leave the bacon grease in the skillet.
4. Add the Brussels sprouts to the bacon grease in the skillet and cook as you stir for about 6 minutes until browned on both side.
5. Push the Brussels sprouts to one side of the skillet, add the whisked eggs and scramble for about 3 to 4 minutes until almost set.
6. Once the bacon is cooled, crumble into small pieces.
7. Divide the Brussels sprouts and scrambled eggs among four serving plates. Scatter the tops with crumbled bacon pieces and garnish with feta cheese before serving.

Per Serving

calories: 255 | fat: 15.3g | protein: 21.3g | carbs: 10.2g | fiber: 4.2g | sugar: 4.2g
sodium: 340mg

Easy and Creamy Grits

Prep time: 5 minutes | Cook time: 10 minutes | Serves 4

- 1 cup fat-free milk

From the Cupboard:
- 2 cups water
- 1 cup stone-ground corn grits

1. Pour the milk and water into a saucepan over medium heat, then bring to a simmer until warmed through.
2. Add the corn grits and stir well. Reduce the heat to low and cook covered for 5 to 7 minutes, whisking continuously, or until the grits become tender.
3. Remove from the heat and serve warm.

Per Serving

calories: 168 | fat: 1.1g | protein: 6.2g | carbs: 33.8g | fiber: 1.1g | sugar: 2.8g
sodium: 33mg

Brussels Sprout with Fried Eggs

Prep time: 10 minutes | Cook time: 15 minutes | Serves 4

- 1 pound (454 g) Brussels sprouts, sliced
- 2 garlic cloves, thinly sliced

From the Cupboard:
- 3 teaspoons extra-virgin olive oil, divided

- Juice of 1 lemon
- 4 eggs

- ¼ teaspoon salt

1. Heat 1½ teaspoons of olive oil in a large skillet over medium heat.
2. Add the Brussels sprouts and sauté for 6 to 8 minutes until crispy and tender, stirring frequently.
3. Stir in the garlic and cook for about 1 minute until fragrant. Sprinkle with the salt and lemon juice.
4. Remove from the skillet to a plate and set aside.
5. Heat the remaining oil in the skillet over medium-high heat. Crack the eggs one at a time into the skillet and fry for about 3 minutes. Flip the eggs and continue cooking, or until the egg whites are set and the yolks are cooked to your liking.
6. Serve the fried eggs over the crispy Brussels sprouts.

Per Serving

calories: 157 | fat: 8.9g | protein: 10.1g | carbs: 11.8g | fiber: 4.1g | sugar: 4.0g
sodium: 233mg

Ham and Jicama Hash

Prep time: 10 minutes | Cook time: 15 minutes | Serves 4

- 6 eggs, beaten
- 2 cups jicama, grated

From the Cupboard:
- Salt and ground black pepper, to taste

- 1 cup low fat Cheddar cheese, grated
- 1 cup ham, diced

- Nonstick cooking spray

1. Spray a large nonstick skillet with cooking spray and place over medium-high heat. Add jicama and cook, stirring occasionally, until it starts to brown, about 5 minutes.
2. Add remaining Ingredients and reduce heat to medium. Cook for about 3 minutes, then flip over and cook until eggs are set, about 3 to 5 minutes more. Season with salt and pepper and serve.

Per Serving

calories: 222 | fat: 11.1g | protein: 21.1g | carbs: 8.2g | fiber: 3.0g | sugar: 2.0g
sodium: 1054mg

Simple Grain-Free Biscuits

Prep time: 10 minutes | Cook time: 15 minutes | Serves 4

- ¼ cup plain low-fat Greek yogurt
- 1½ cups finely ground almond flour

From the Cupboard:
- 2 tablespoons unsalted butter
- Pinch salt

1. Preheat the oven to 375ºF (190ºC). Line a baking sheet with parchment paper and set aside.
2. Place the butter in a microwave-safe bowl and microwave for 15 to 20 seconds, or until it is just enough to soften.
3. Add the yogurt and salt to the bowl of butter and blend well.
4. Slowly pour in the almond flour and keep stirring until the mixture just comes together into a slightly sticky, shaggy dough.
5. Use a ¼-cup measuring cup to mound balls of dough onto the parchment-lined baking sheet and flatten each into a rounded biscuit shape, about 1 inch thick.
6. Bake in the preheated oven for 13 to 15 minutes, or until the biscuits are lightly golden brown.
7. Let the biscuits cool for 5 minutes before serving.

Per Serving

calories: 309 | fat: 28.1g | protein: 9.9g | carbs: 8.7g | fiber: 5.1g | sugar: 2.0g
sodium: 31mg

Peanut Butter and Berry Oatmeal

Prep time: 5 minutes | Cook time: 5 minutes | Serves 2

- 1½ cups unsweetened vanilla almond milk
- ¾ cup rolled oats
- 1 tablespoon chia seeds
- 2 tablespoons natural peanut butter
- ¼ cup fresh berries, divided (optional)

1. Add the almond milk, oats, and chia seeds to a small saucepan and bring to a boil.
2. Cover and continue cooking, stirring often, or until the oats have absorbed the milk.
3. Add the peanut butter and keep stirring until the oats are thick and creamy.
4. Divide the oatmeal into two serving bowls. Serve topped with the berries.

Per Serving

calories: 260 | fat: 13.9g | protein: 10.1g | carbs: 26.9g | fiber: 7.1g | sugar: 1.0g
sodium: 130mg

Scrambled Egg Whites with Bell Pepper

Prep time: 5 minutes | Cook time: 10 minutes | Serves 2

- 1 green bell pepper, deseeded and finely chopped
- ½ red onion, finely chopped

From the Cupboard:

- 2 tablespoons extra-virgin olive oil

- 4 eggs whites
- 2 ounces (57 g) pepper Jack cheese, grated

- ½ teaspoon sea salt

1. Heat the olive oil in a nonstick skillet over medium-high heat..
2. Add the bell pepper and onion to the skillet and sauté for 5 minutes or until tender.
3. Sprinkle the egg white with salt in a bowl, then pour the egg whites in the skillet. Cook for 3 minutes or until the egg whites are scrambled. Stir the egg whites halfway through.
4. Scatter with cheese and cook for an additional 1 minutes until the cheese melts.
5. Divide them onto two serving plates and serve warm.

Per Serving

calories: 316 | fat: 23.3g | protein: 22.3g | carbs: 6.2g | fiber: 1.1g | sugar: 4.2g
sodium: 975mg

Berry Bark

Prep time: 10 minutes | Cook time: 0 minutes | Serves 6

- 3 to 4 strawberries, sliced
- 1½ cup plain Greek yogurt
- ½ cup blueberries

- ½ cup low fat granola
- 3 tablespoons sugar free maple syrup

1. Line a baking sheet with parchment paper.
2. In a medium bowl, mix yogurt and syrup until combined. Pour into prepared pan and spread in a thin even layer.
3. Top with remaining Ingredients. Cover with foil and freeze two hours or overnight.
4. Slice into squares and serve immediately. If bark thaws too much it will lose its shape. Store any remaining bark in an airtight container in the freezer.

Per Serving

calories: 70 | fat: 6.0g | protein: 7.1g | carbs: 18.2g | fiber: 1.9g | sugar: 7.1g
sodium: 22mg

Cauliflower Hash

Prep time: 10 minutes | Cook time: 20 minutes | Serves 2

- 4 cups cauliflower, grated
- 1 cup mushrooms, diced
- ¾ cup onion, diced
- 3 slices bacon
- ¼ cup sharp Cheddar cheese, grated

1. In a medium skillet, over medium-high heat, fry bacon, set aside.
2. Add vegetables to the skillet and cook, stirring occasionally, until golden brown.
3. Cut bacon into pieces and return to skillet.
4. Top with cheese and allow it to melt. Serve immediately.

Per Serving

calories: 156 | fat: 6.9g | protein: 10.1g | carbs: 16.2g | fiber: 5.9g | sugar: 7.1g
sodium: 358mg

Goat Cheese and Avocado Toast

Prep time: 10 minutes | Cook time: 5 minutes | Serves 2

- 2 slices whole-wheat bread, thinly sliced
- ½ avocado

From the Cupboard:
- Salt, to taste

- 2 tablespoons goat cheese, crumbled
- 2 slices of crumbled bacon, for topping (optional)

1. Toast the bread slices in a toaster for 2 to 3 minutes on each side until golden brown.
2. Using a large spoon, scoop the avocado flesh out of the skin and transfer to a medium bowl. Mash the flesh with a potato masher or the back of a fork until it has a spreadable consistency.
3. Spoon the mashed avocado onto the bread slices and evenly spread it all over.
4. Scatter with crumbled goat cheese and lightly season with salt.
5. Serve topped with crumbled bacon, if desired.

Per Serving

calories: 140 | fat: 6.2g | protein: 5.2g | carbs: 18.2g | fiber: 5.1g | sugar: 0g
sodium: 197mg

Coconut Porridge

Prep time: 2 minutes | Cook time: 10 minutes | Serves 4

- 4 cup vanilla almond milk, unsweetened
- 1 cup unsweetened coconut, grated
- 8 teaspoons coconut flour

1. Add coconut to a saucepan and cook over medium-high heat until it is lightly toasted. Be careful not to let it burn.
2. Add milk and bring to a boil. While stirring, slowly add flour, cook and stir until mixture starts to thicken, about 5 minutes.
3. Remove from heat, mixture will thicken more as it cools. Ladle into bowls, add blueberries, or drizzle with a little honey if desired.

Per Serving

calories: 233 | fat: 13.9g | protein: 6.1g | carbs: 21.2g | fiber: 12.9g | sugar: 4.1g
sodium: 289mg

Easy Turkey Breakfast Patties

Prep time: 10 minutes | Cook time: 10 minutes | Serves 8 (1 patty each)

- 1 pound (454 g) lean ground turkey
- ½ teaspoon dried thyme

From the Cupboard:

- ½ teaspoon salt
- ½ teaspoon freshly ground black

- ½ teaspoon dried sage
- ¼ teaspoon ground fennel seeds

pepper
- 1 teaspoon extra-virgin olive oil

1. Mix the ground turkey, thyme, sage, salt, pepper, and fennel in a large bowl, and stir until well combined.
2. Form the turkey mixture into 8 equal-sized patties with your hands.
3. In a skillet, heat the olive oil over medium-high heat. Cook the patties for 3 to 4 minutes per side until cooked through.
4. Transfer the patties to a plate and serve hot.

Per Serving

calories: 91 | fat: 4.8g | protein: 11.2g | carbs: 0.1g | fiber: 0.1g | sugar: 0g
sodium: 155mg

CHAPTER 5

LUNCH

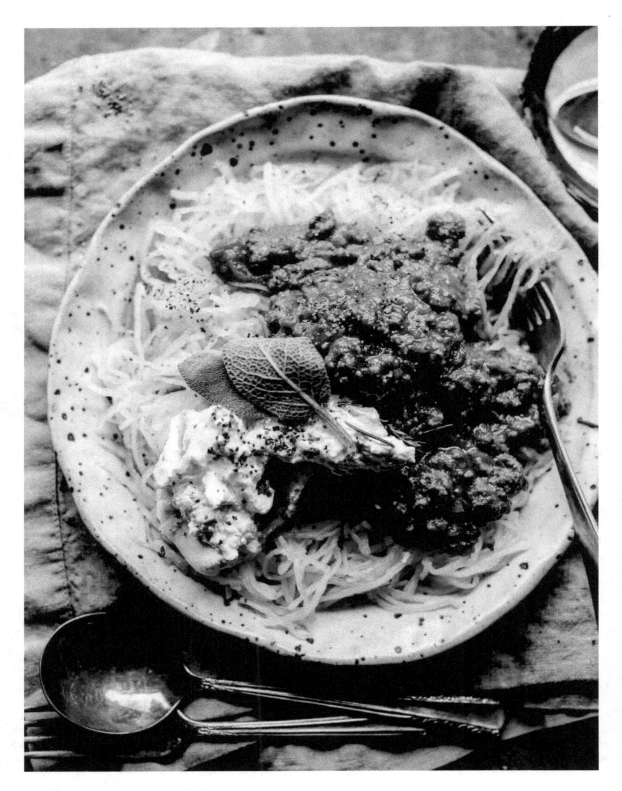

Spaghetti Squash and Chickpea Bolognese

Prep time: 5 minutes | Cook time: 25 minutes | Serves 4

- 1 (3- to 4-pound / 1.4- to 1.8-kg) spaghetti squash
- ½ teaspoon ground cumin
- 1 cup no-sugar-added spaghetti sauce
- 1 (15-ounce / 425-g) can low-sodium chickpeas, drained and rinsed
- 6 ounces (170 g) extra-firm tofu

1. Preheat the oven to 400°F (205°C).
2. Cut the squash in half lengthwise. Scoop out the seeds and discard.
3. Season both halves of the squash with the cumin, and place them on a baking sheet cut-side down. Roast for 25 minutes.
4. Meanwhile, heat a medium saucepan over low heat, and pour in the spaghetti sauce and chickpeas.
5. Press the tofu between two layers of paper towels, and gently squeeze out any excess water.
6. Crumble the tofu into the sauce and cook for 15 minutes.
7. Remove the squash from the oven, and comb through the flesh of each half with a fork to make thin strands.
8. Divide the "spaghetti" into four portions, and top each portion with one-quarter of the sauce.

Per Serving

calories: 276 | fat: 7.1g | protein: 14.1g | carbs: 41.9g | fiber: 10.1g | sugar: 7.0g
sodium: 56mg

Eggplant-Zucchini Parmesan

Prep time: 10 minutes | Cook time: 2 hours | Serves 6

- 1 medium eggplant, peeled and cut into 1-inch cubes
- 1 medium zucchini, cut into 1-inch pieces
- 1 medium onion, cut into thin wedges
- 1½ cups purchased light spaghetti sauce
- ⅔ cup reduced fat Parmesan cheese, grated

1. Place the vegetables, spaghetti sauce and ⅓ cup Parmesan in the crock pot. Stir to combine. Cover and cook on high for 2 to 2 ½ hours, or on low 4 to 5 hours.
2. Sprinkle remaining Parmesan on top before serving.

Per Serving

calories: 82 | fat: 2.0g | protein: 5.1g | carbs: 12.1g | fiber: 5.0g | sugar: 7.0g
sodium: 456mg

Grilled Portobello and Zucchini Burger

Prep time: 5 minutes | Cook time: 10 minutes | Serves 2

- 2 large portabella mushroom caps
- ½ small zucchini, sliced
- 2 slices low fat cheese

From the Cupboard:
- 2 teaspoons olive oil

- 2 whole wheat sandwich thins
- 2 teaspoons roasted red bell peppers

1. Heat grill, or charcoal, to medium-high heat.
2. Lightly brush mushroom caps with olive oil. Grill mushroom caps and zucchini slices until tender, about 3 to 4 minutes per side.
3. Place on sandwich thin. Top with sliced cheese and roasted red bell pepper. Serve.

Per Serving

calories: 178 | fat: 3.0g | protein: 15.1g | carbs: 26.1g | fiber: 8.0g | sugar: 3.0g
sodium: 520mg

Pulled Pork Sandwiches with Apricot Jelly

Prep time: 5 minutes | Cook time: 15 minutes | Serves 4

- 8 ounces (227 g) store-bought pulled pork
- ½ cup chopped green bell pepper

From the Cupboard:
- Avocado oil cooking spray

- 2 slices provolone cheese
- 4 whole-wheat sandwich thins
- 2½ tablespoons apricot jelly

1. Heat the pulled pork according to the package instructions.
2. Heat a medium skillet over medium-low heat. When hot, coat the cooking surface with cooking spray.
3. Put the bell pepper in the skillet and cook for 5 minutes. Transfer to a small bowl and set aside.
4. Meanwhile, tear each slice of cheese into 2 strips, and halve the sandwich thins so you have a top and bottom.
5. Reduce the heat to low, and place the sandwich thins in the skillet cut-side down to toast, about 2 minutes.
6. Remove the sandwich thins from the skillet. Spread one-quarter of the jelly on the bottom half of each sandwich thin, then place one-quarter of the cheese, pulled pork, and pepper on top. Cover with the top half of the sandwich thin.

Per Serving

calories: 250 | fat: 8.1g | protein: 16.1g | carbs: 34.1g | fiber: 6.1g | sugar: 8.0g
sodium: 510mg

Wilted Dandelion Greens with Sweet Onion

Prep time: 15 minutes | Cook time: 12 minutes | Serves 4

- 1 Vidalia onion, thinly sliced
- 2 garlic cloves, minced
- 2 bunches dandelion greens, roughly chopped
- ½ cup low-sodium vegetable broth
- From the Cupboard:
- 1 tablespoon extra-virgin olive oil
- Freshly ground black pepper, to taste

1. Heat the olive oil in a large skillet over low heat.
2. Cook the onion and garlic for 2 to 3 minutes until tender, stirring occasionally.
3. Add the dandelion greens and broth and cook for 5 to 7 minutes, stirring frequently, or until the greens are wilted.
4. Transfer to a plate and season with black pepper. Serve warm.

Per Serving

calories: 81 | fat: 3.8g | protein: 3.1g | carbs: 10.7g | fiber: 3.8g | sugar: 2.0g
sodium: 72mg

Simple Buttercup Squash Soup

Prep time: 15 minutes | Cook time: 33 minutes | Serves 6

- 1 medium onion, chopped
- 1½ pounds (680 g) buttercup squash, peeled, deseeded, and cut into 1-inch chunks
- 4 cups vegetable broth
- Ground nutmeg, to taste

From the Cupboard:

- 2 tablespoons extra-virgin olive oil
- ½ teaspoon kosher salt
- ¼ teaspoon ground white pepper

1. Heat the olive oil in a pot over medium-high heat until shimmering.
2. Add the onion and sauté for 3 minutes or until translucent.
3. Add the buttercup squash, vegetable broth, salt, and pepper. Stir to mix well. Bring to a boil.
4. Reduce the heat to low and simmer for 30 minutes or until the buttercup squash is soft.
5. Pour the soup in a food processor, then pulse to purée until creamy and smooth.
6. Pour the soup in a large serving bowl, then sprinkle with ground nutmeg and serve.

Per Serving (1⅓ Cups)

calories: 110 | fat: 5.0g | protein: 1.0g | carbs: 18.0g | fiber: 4.0g | sugar: 4.0g
sodium: 166mg

Lemon Parsley White Fish Fillets

- 4 (6-ounce / 170-g) lean white fish fillets, rinsed and patted dry
- 2 tablespoons parsley, finely chopped

From the Cupboard:

- Cooking spray
- Paprika, to taste

- ½ teaspoon lemon zest
- ¼ teaspoon dried dill
- 1 medium lemon, halved

- Salt and pepper, to taste
- ¼ cup extra virgin olive oil

1. Preheat the oven to 400ºF (205ºC). Line a baking sheet with aluminum foil and spray with cooking spray.
2. Place the fillets on the foil and scatter with the paprika. Season as desired with salt and pepper.
3. Bake in the preheated oven for 10 minutes, or until the flesh flakes easily with a fork.
4. Meanwhile, stir together the parsley, lemon zest, olive oil, and dill in a small bowl.
5. Remove the fish from the oven to four plates. Squeeze the lemon juice over the fish and serve topped with the parsley mixture.

Per Serving

calories: 283 | fat: 17.2g | protein: 33.3g | carbs: 1.0g | fiber: 0g | sugar: 0g
sodium: 74mg

Lemon Wax Beans

- 2 pounds (907 g) wax beans
- Juice of ½ lemon
- From the Cupboard:

- 2 tablespoons extra-virgin olive oil
- Sea salt and freshly ground black pepper, to taste

1. Preheat the oven to 400ºF (205ºC).
2. Line a baking sheet with aluminum foil.
3. In a large bowl, toss the beans and olive oil. Season lightly with salt and pepper.
4. Transfer the beans to the baking sheet and spread them out.
5. Roast the beans until caramelized and tender, about 10 to 12 minutes.
6. Transfer the beans to a serving platter and sprinkle with the lemon juice.

Per Serving

calories: 99 | fat: 7.1g | protein: 2.1g | carbs: 8.1g | fiber: 4.2g | sugar: 3.9g
sodium: 814mg

Cilantro Lime Shrimp

Prep time: 15 minutes | Cook time: 8 minutes | Serves 4

- ½ teaspoon garlic clove, minced
- 1 pound (454 g) large shrimp, peeled and deveined

From the Cupboard:

- 1 teaspoon extra virgin olive oil
- ¼ teaspoon salt

- ¼ cup chopped fresh cilantro, or more to taste
- 1 lime, zested and juiced

- ⅛ teaspoon black pepper

1. In a large heavy skillet, heat the olive oil over medium-high heat.
2. Add the minced garlic and cook for 30 seconds until fragrant.
3. Toss in the shrimp and cook for about 5 to 6 minutes, stirring occasionally, or until they turn pink and opaque.
4. Remove from the heat to a bowl. Add the cilantro, lime zest and juice, salt, and pepper to the shrimp, and toss to combine. Serve immediately.

Per Serving

calories: 133 | fat: 3.5g | protein: 24.3g | carbs: 1.0g | fiber: 0g | sugar: 0g
sodium: 258mg

Butter Cod with Asparagus

Prep time: 5 minutes | Cook time: 10 minutes | Serves 4

- 4 (4-ounce / 113-g) cod fillets
- ¼ teaspoon garlic powder
- 24 asparagus spears, woody ends trimmed

From the Cupboard:

- ¼ teaspoon salt
- ¼ teaspoon freshly ground black

- ½ cup brown rice, cooked
- 1 tablespoon freshly squeezed lemon juice

- pepper
- 2 tablespoons unsalted butter

1. In a large bowl, season the cod fillets with the garlic powder, salt, and pepper. Set aside.
2. Melt the butter in a skillet over medium-low heat.
3. Place the cod fillets and asparagus in the skillet in a single layer. Cook covered for 8 minutes, or until the cod is cooked through.
4. Divide the cooked brown rice, cod fillets, and asparagus among four plates. Serve drizzled with the lemon juice.

Per Serving

calories: 233 | fat: 8.2g | protein: 22.1g | carbs: 20.1g | fiber: 5.2g | sugar: 2.2g
sodium: 275mg

Cajun Catfish

- 4 (8-ounce / 227-g) catfish fillets
- 2 teaspoons thyme

From the Cupboard:
- 2 tablespoons olive oil
- 2 teaspoons garlic salt
- 2 teaspoons paprika

- ½ teaspoon red hot sauce

- ½ teaspoon cayenne pepper
- ¼ teaspoon black pepper
- Nonstick cooking spray

1. Heat oven to 450ºF (235ºC). Spray a baking dish with cooking spray.
2. In a small bowl whisk together everything but catfish. Brush both sides of fillets, using all the spice mix.
3. Bake 10 to 13 minutes or until fish flakes easily with a fork. Serve.

Per Serving

calories: 367 | fat: 24.0g | protein: 35.2g | carbs: 0g | fiber: 0g | sugar: 0g
sodium: 70mg

Lamb and Mushroom CheeseBurgers

- 8 ounces (227 g) grass-fed ground lamb
- 8 ounces (227 g) brown mushrooms,

From the Cupboard:
- ¼ teaspoon salt
- ¼ teaspoon freshly ground black pepper

finely chopped
- ¼ cup crumbled goat cheese
- 1 tablespoon minced fresh basil

1. In a large mixing bowl, combine the lamb, mushrooms, salt, and pepper, and mix well.
2. In a small bowl, mix the goat cheese and basil.
3. Form the lamb mixture into 4 patties, reserving about ½ cup of the mixture in the bowl. In each patty, make an indentation in the center and fill with 1 tablespoon of the goat cheese mixture. Use the reserved meat mixture to close the burgers. Press the meat firmly to hold together.
4. Heat the barbecue or a large skillet over medium-high heat. Add the burgers and cook for 5 to 7 minutes on each side, until cooked through. Serve.

Per Serving

calories: 172 | fat: 13.1g | protein: 11.1g | carbs: 2.9g | fiber: 0g | sugar: 1.0g
sodium: 155mg

Parmesan Golden Pork Chops

Prep time: 10 minutes | Cook time: 25 minutes | Serves 4

- 4 bone-in, thin-cut pork chops
- ½ cup grated Parmesan cheese

From the Cupboard:
- Nonstick cooking spray
- 2 tablespoons butter

- 3 garlic cloves, minced
- ¼ teaspoon dried thyme

- ¼ teaspoon salt
- Freshly ground black pepper, to taste

1. Preheat the oven to 400ºF (205ºC). Line a baking sheet with parchment paper and spray with nonstick cooking spray.
2. Arrange the pork chops on the prepared baking sheet so they do not overlap.
3. In a small bowl, combine the butter, cheese, garlic, salt, thyme, and pepper. Press 2 tablespoons of the cheese mixture onto the top of each pork chop.
4. Bake for 18 to 22 minutes until the pork is cooked through and its juices run clear. Set the broiler to high, then broil for 1 to 2 minutes to brown the tops.

Per Serving

calories: 333 | fat: 16.1g | protein: 44.1g | carbs: 1.1g | fiber: 0g | sugar: 0g
sodium: 441mg

Chipotle Chili Pork

Prep time: 4 hours 20 minutes | Cook time: 20 minutes | Serves 4

- 4 (5-ounce / 142-g) pork chops, about 1 inch thick
- 1 tablespoon chipotle chili powder

From the Cupboard:
- 1 tablespoon extra-virgin olive oil

- Juice and zest of 1 lime
- 2 teaspoons minced garlic
- 1 teaspoon ground cinnamon

- Pinch sea salt

1. Combine all the ingredients, except for the lemon wedges, in a large bowl. Toss to combine well.
2. Wrap the bowl in plastic and refrigerate to marinate for at least 4 hours.
3. Preheat the oven to 400ºF (205ºC). Set a rack on a baking sheet.
4. Remove the bowl from the refrigerator and let sit for 15 minutes. Discard the marinade and place the pork on the rack.
5. Roast in the preheated oven for 20 minutes or until well browned. Flip the pork halfway through the cooking time.
6. Serve immediately.

Per Serving

calories: 204 | fat: 9.0g | protein: 30.0g | carbs: 1.0g | fiber: 0g | sugar: 1.0g
sodium: 317mg

Butter-Lemon Grilled Cod on Asparagus

Prep time: 5 minutes | Cook time: 9 to 12 minutes | Serves 4

- 1 pound (454 g) asparagus spears, ends trimmed
- 4 (4-ounce / 113-g) cod fillets, rinsed

and patted dry
- Juice and zest of 1 medium lemon

From the Cupboard:

- Cooking spray
- ¼ teaspoon black pepper (optional)
- ¼ cup light butter with canola oil
- ¼ teaspoon salt (optional)

1. Heat a grill pan over medium-high heat.
2. Spray the asparagus spears with cooking spray. Cook the asparagus for 6 to 8 minutes until fork-tender, flipping occasionally.
3. Transfer to a large platter and keep warm.
4. Spray both sides of fillets with cooking spray. Season with ¼ teaspoon black pepper, if needed. Add the fillets to the pan and sear each side for 3 minutes until opaque.
5. Meantime, in a small bowl, whisk together the light butter, lemon zest, and ¼ teaspoon salt (if desired).
6. Spoon and spread the mixture all over the asparagus. Place the fish on top and squeeze the lemon juice over the fish. Serve immediately.

Per Serving

calories: 158 | fat: 6.4g | protein: 23.0g | carbs: 6.1g | fiber: 3.0g | sugar: 2.8g
sodium: 212mg

Zucchini and Pinto Bean Casserole

Prep time: 15 minutes | Cook time: 15 minutes | Serves 4

- 1 (6 to 7-inch) zucchini, trimmed
- 1 (15-ounce / 425-g) can pinto beans or 1½ cups Salt-Free No-Soak Beans, rinsed and drained
- 1⅓ cups salsa
- 1⅓ cups shredded Mexican cheese blend

From the Cupboard:

- Nonstick cooking spray

1. Slice the zucchini into rounds. You'll need at least 16 slices.
2. Spray a 6-inch cake pan with nonstick spray.
3. Put the beans into a medium bowl and mash some of them with a fork.
4. Cover the bottom of the pan with about 4 zucchini slices. Add about ⅓ of the beans, ⅓ cup of salsa, and ⅓ cup of cheese. Press down. Repeat for 2 more layers. Add the remaining zucchini, salsa, and cheese. (There are no beans in the top layer.)
5. Cover the pan loosely with foil.

6. Pour 1 cup of water into the electric pressure cooker.
7. Place the pan on the wire rack and carefully lower it into the pot. Close and lock the lid of the pressure cooker. Set the valve to sealing.
8. Cook on high pressure for 15 minutes.
9. When the cooking is complete, hit Cancel and allow the pressure to release naturally.
10. Once the pin drops, unlock and remove the lid.
11. Carefully remove the pan from the pot, lifting by the handles of the wire rack. Let the casserole sit for 5 minutes before slicing into quarters and serving.

Per Serving

calories: 251 | fat: 12.1g | protein: 16.1g | carbs: 22.9g | fiber: 7.1g | sugar: 4.0g
sodium: 1080mg

Asparagus and Scallop Skillet with Lemony

Prep time: 10 minutes | Cook time: 15 minutes | Serves 4

- 1 pound (454 g) asparagus, trimmed and cut into 2-inch segments
- 1 pound (454 g) sea scallops

From the Cupboard:
- 3 teaspoons extra-virgin olive oil, divided
- 1 tablespoon butter

- ¼ cup dry white wine
- 2 garlic cloves, minced
- Juice of 1 lemon

- ¼ teaspoon freshly ground black pepper

1. Heat half of olive oil in a nonstick skillet over medium heat until shimmering.
2. Add the asparagus to the skillet and sauté for 6 minutes until soft. Transfer the cooked asparagus to a large plate and cover with aluminum foil.
3. Heat the remaining half of olive oil and butter in the skillet until the butter is melted.
4. Add the scallops to the skillet and cook for 6 minutes or until opaque and browned. Flip the scallops with tongs halfway through the cooking time. Transfer the scallops to the plate and cover with aluminum foil.
5. Combine the wine, garlic, lemon juice, and black pepper in the skillet. Simmer over medium-low heat for 2 minutes. Keep stirring during the simmering.
6. Pour the sauce over the asparagus and scallops to coat well, then serve warm.

Per Serving

calories: 256 | fat: 6.9g | protein: 26.1g | carbs: 14.9g | fiber: 2.1g | sugar: 2.9g
sodium: 491mg

Leek and Cauliflower Soup

Prep time: 10 minutes | Cook time: 20 minutes | Serves 2

- 2½ cups chopped leeks (2 to 3 leeks)
- 2½ cups cauliflower florets
- 1 garlic clove, peeled

From the Cupboard:

- Avocado oil cooking spray
- ¼ teaspoon salt

- $^{1}/_{3}$ cup low-sodium vegetable broth
- ½ cup half-and-half

- ¼ teaspoon freshly ground black pepper

1. Heat a large stockpot over medium-low heat. When hot, coat the cooking surface with cooking spray. Put the leeks and cauliflower into the pot.
2. Increase the heat to medium and cover the pan. Cook for 10 minutes, stirring halfway through.
3. Add the garlic and cook for 5 minutes.
4. Add the broth and deglaze the pan, stirring to scrape up the browned bits from the bottom.
5. Transfer the broth and vegetables to a food processor or blender and add the half-and-half, salt, and pepper. Blend well.

Per Serving

calories: 174 | fat: 7.1g | protein: 6.1g | carbs: 23.9g | fiber: 5.1g | sugar: 8.0g
sodium: 490mg

Asparagus with Scallops

Prep time: 10 minutes | Cook time: 15 minutes | Serves 4

- 1 pound (454 g) asparagus, trimmed and cut into 2-inch segments
- 1 pound (454 g) sea scallops

From the Cupboard:

- 3 teaspoons extra-virgin olive oil, divided
- 1 tablespoon butter

- ¼ cup dry white wine
- Juice of 1 lemon
- 2 garlic cloves, minced

- ¼ teaspoon freshly ground black pepper

1. In a large skillet, heat 1½ teaspoons of oil over medium heat.
2. Add the asparagus and sauté for 5 to 6 minutes until just tender, stirring regularly. Remove from the skillet and cover with aluminum foil to keep warm.
3. Add the remaining 1½ teaspoons of oil and the butter to the skillet. When the butter is melted and sizzling, place the scallops in a single layer in the skillet. Cook for about 3 minutes on one side until nicely browned. Use tongs to gently loosen and flip the scallops, and cook on the other side for another 3 minutes until browned and cooked through. Remove and cover with foil to keep warm.

4. In the same skillet, combine the wine, lemon juice, garlic, and pepper. Bring to a simmer for 1 to 2 minutes, stirring to mix in any browned pieces left in the pan.
5. Return the asparagus and the cooked scallops to the skillet to coat with the sauce. Serve warm.

Per Serving

calories: 253 | fat: 7.1g | protein: 26.1g | carbs: 14.9g | fiber: 2.1g | sugar: 3.1g
sodium: 494mg

Creamy Cod Fillet with Quinoa and Asparagus

Prep time: 5 minutes | Cook time: 15 minutes | Serves 4

- ½ cup uncooked quinoa
- 4 (4-ounce / 113-g) cod fillets
- ½ teaspoon garlic powder, divided

From the Cupboard:

- ¼ teaspoon salt
- ¼ teaspoon freshly ground black

- 24 asparagus spears, cut the bottom 1½ inches off
- 1 cup half-and-half

  pepper
- 1 tablespoon avocado oil

1. Put the quinoa in a pot of salted water. Bring to a boil. Reduce the heat to low and simmer for 15 minutes or until the quinoa is soft and has a white "tail". Cover and turn off the heat. Let sit for 5 minutes.
2. On a clean work surface, rub the cod fillets with ¼ teaspoon of garlic powder, salt, and pepper.
3. Heat the avocado oil in a nonstick skillet over medium-low heat.
4. Add the cod fillets and asparagus in the skillet and cook for 8 minutes or until they are tender. Flip the cod and shake the skillet halfway through the cooking time.
5. Pour the half-and-half in the skillet, and sprinkle with remaining garlic powder. Turn up the heat to high and simmer for 2 minutes until creamy.
6. Divide the quinoa, cod fillets, and asparagus in four bowls and serve warm.

Per Serving

calories: 258 | fat: 7.9g | protein: 25.2g | carbs: 22.7g | fiber: 5.2g | sugar: 3.8g
sodium: 410mg

CHAPTER 6

DINNER

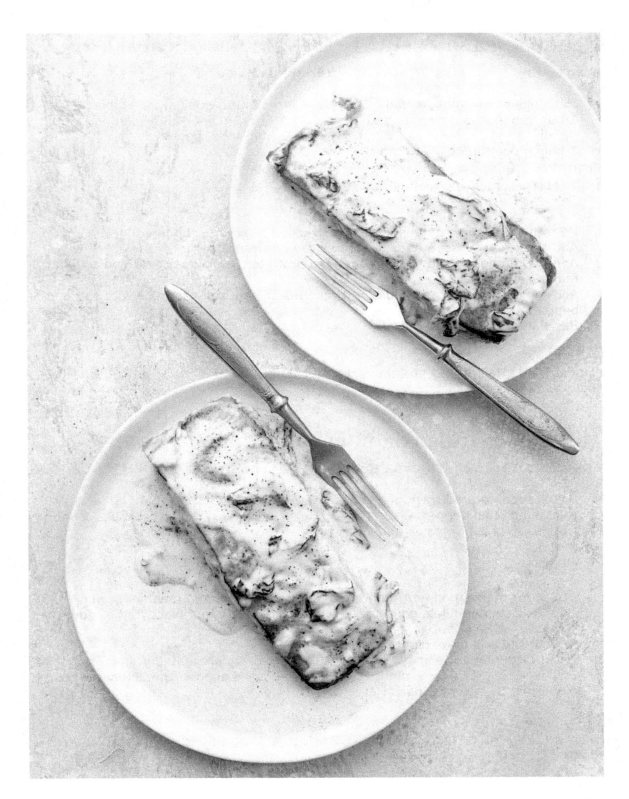

Dandelion and Beet Greens with Black Beans

Prep time: 10 minutes | Cook time: 15 minutes | Serves 4

- ½ Vidalia onion, thinly sliced
- 1 bunch dandelion greens, cut into ribbons
- 1 bunch beet greens, cut into ribbons

From the Cupboard:

- 1 tablespoon olive oil
- Salt and freshly ground black pepper,

- ½ cup low-sodium vegetable broth
- 1 (15-ounce / 425-g) can no-salt-added black beans

to taste

1. Heat the olive oil in a nonstick skillet over low heat until shimmering.
2. Add the onion and sauté for 3 minutes or until translucent.
3. Add the dandelion and beet greens, and broth to the skillet. Cover and cook for 8 minutes or until wilted.
4. Add the black beans and cook for 4 minutes or until soft. Sprinkle with salt and pepper. Stir to mix well.
5. Serve immediately.

Per Serving

calories: 161 | fat: 4.0g | protein: 9.0g | carbs: 26.0g | fiber: 10.0g | sugar: 1.0g
sodium: 224mg

Marinated Grilled Salmon with Lemongrass

Prep time: 10 minutes | Cook time: 8 to 12 minutes | Serves 4

- 1 tablespoon grated fresh ginger
- 1 small hot chili pepper
- 1 tablespoon lemongrass, minced

From the Cupboard:

- 1 tablespoon olive oil

- 1 tablespoon Splenda
- 4 (4-ounce / 113-g) skinless salmon fillets

- 2 tablespoons low-sodium soy sauce

1. Except for the salmon, stir together all the ingredients in a medium bowl. Brush the salmon fillets generously with the marinade and place in the fridge to marinate for 30 minutes.
2. Preheat the grill to medium heat.
3. Discard the marinade and transfer the salmon to the preheated grill.
4. Grill each side for 4 to 6 minutes, or until the fish is almost completely cooked through at the thickest part. Serve hot.

Per Serving

calories: 223 | fat: 12.2g | protein: 25.7g | carbs: 2.0g | fiber: 0g | sugar: 2.9g
sodium: 203mg

Cheesy Mushroom and Pesto Flatbreads

Prep time: 5 minutes | Cook time: 13 to 17 minutes | Serves 2

- ½ red onion, sliced
- ½ cup sliced mushrooms
- ¼ cup store-bought pesto sauce

From the Cupboard:

- 1 teaspoon extra-virgin olive oil
- Salt and freshly ground black pepper, to taste

- 2 whole-wheat flatbreads
- ¼ cup shredded Mozzarella cheese

1. Preheat the oven to 350°F (180°C).
2. Heat the olive oil in a small skillet over medium heat. Add the onion slices and mushrooms to the skillet, and sauté for 3 to 5 minutes, stirring occasionally, or until they start to soften. Season with salt and pepper.
3. Meanwhile, spoon 2 tablespoons of pesto sauce onto each flatbread and spread it all over. Evenly divide the mushroom mixture between two flatbreads, then scatter each top with 2 tablespoons of shredded cheese.
4. Transfer the flatbreads to a baking sheet and bake until the cheese melts and bubbles, about 10 to 12 minutes.
5. Let the flatbreads cool for 5 minutes and serve warm.

Per Serving

calories: 346 | fat: 22.8g | protein: 14.2g | carbs: 27.6g | fiber: 7.3g | sugar: 4.0g
sodium: 790mg

Fried Rice with Snap Peas

Prep time: 5 minutes | Cook time: 15 minutes | Serves 8

- 2 cups sugar snap peas
- 2 egg whites
- 1 egg

From the Cupboard:

- 2 tablespoons lite soy sauce

- 1 cup instant brown rice, cooked according to directions

1. Add the peas to the cooked rice and mix to combine.
2. In a small skillet, scramble the egg and egg whites. Add the rice and peas to the skillet and stir in soy sauce. Cook, stirring frequently, about 2 to 3 minutes, or until heated through. Serve.

Per Serving

calories: 108 | fat: 1.0g | protein: 4.1g | carbs: 20.1g | fiber: 1.0g | sugar: 1.0g
sodium: 151mg

Chili Relleno Casserole

Prep time: 5 minutes | Cook time: 35 minutes | Serves 8

- 3 eggs
- 1 cup Monterey jack pepper cheese, grated
- ¾ cup half-and-half
- ½ cup Cheddar cheese, grated
- 2 (7-ounce / 198-g) cans whole green chilies, drain well

From the Cupboard:

- ½ teaspoon salt
- Nonstick cooking spray

1. Heat oven to 350ºF (180ºC). Spray a baking pan with cooking spray.
2. Slice each chili down one long side and lay flat.
3. Arrange half the chilies in the prepared baking pan, skin side down, in single layer.
4. Sprinkle with the pepper cheese and top with remaining chilies, skin side up.
5. In a small bowl, beat eggs, salt, and half-and-half. Pour over chilies. Top with Cheddar cheese.
6. Bake 35 minutes, or until top is golden brown. Let rest 10 minutes before serving.

Per Serving

calories: 296 | fat: 13.0g | protein: 13.1g | carbs: 36.1g | fiber: 14.0g | sugar:21.0g sodium: 463mg

Sautéed Zucchini and Tomatoes

Prep time: 10 minutes | Cook time: 10 minutes | Serves 4

- 1 sliced onion
- 2 pounds (907 g) zucchini, peeled and cut into 1-inch-thick slices
- 2 tomatoes, chopped
- 1 green bell pepper, chopped

From the Cupboard:

- 1 tablespoon vegetable oil
- Salt and freshly ground black pepper, to taste

1. Heat the vegetable oil in a nonstick skillet until it shimmers.
2. Sauté the onion slices in the oil for about 3 minutes until translucent, stirring occasionally.
3. Add the zucchini, tomatoes, bell pepper, salt, and pepper to the skillet and stir to combine.
4. Reduce the heat, cover, and continue cooking for about 5 minutes, or until the veggies are tender.
5. Remove from the heat to a large plate and serve hot.

Per Serving

calories: 110 | fat: 4.4g | protein: 6.9g | carbs: 10.7g | fiber: 3.4g | sugar: 2.2g sodium: 11mg

Green Salmon Florentine

Prep time: 10 minutes | Cook time: 30 minutes | Serves 4

- ½ sweet onion, finely chopped
- 1 teaspoon minced garlic
- 3 cups baby spinach

From the Cupboard:

- 1 teaspoon extra-virgin olive oil
- Sea salt and freshly ground black pepper, to taste

- 1 cup kale, tough stems removed, torn into 3-inch pieces
- 4 (5-ounce / 142-g) salmon fillets

1. Preheat the oven to 350ºF (180ºC).
2. Place a large skillet over medium-high heat and add the oil.
3. Sauté the onion and garlic until softened and translucent, about 3 minutes.
4. Add the spinach and kale and sauté until the greens wilt, about 5 minutes.
5. Remove the skillet from the heat and season the greens with salt and pepper.
6. Place the salmon fillets so they are nestled in the greens and partially covered by them. Bake the salmon until it is opaque, about 20 minutes.
7. Serve immediately.

Per Serving

calories: 282 | fat: 15.9g | protein: 28.9g | carbs: 4.1g | fiber: 1.1g | sugar: 0.9g
sodium: 92mg

Fresh Rosemary Trout

Prep time: 5 minutes | Cook time: 7 to 8 minutes | Serves 2

- 4 to 6 fresh rosemary sprigs
- 8 ounces (227 g) trout fillets, about ¼

From the Cupboard:

- ½ teaspoon olive oil
- ⅛ teaspoon salt

inch thick; rinsed and patted dry
- 1 teaspoon fresh lemon juice

- ⅛ teaspoon ground black pepper

1. Preheat the oven to 350ºF (180ºC).
2. Put the rosemary sprigs in a small baking pan in a single row. Spread the fillets on the top of the rosemary sprigs.
3. Brush both sides of each piece of fish with the olive oil. Sprinkle with the salt, pepper, and lemon juice.
4. Bake in the preheated oven for 7 to 8 minutes, or until the fish is opaque and flakes easily.
5. Divide the fillets between two plates and serve hot.

Per Serving

calories: 180 | fat: 9.1g | protein: 23.8g | carbs: 0g | fiber: 0g | sugar: 0g
sodium: 210mg

Grilled Shrimp Skewers

Prep time: 10 minutes | Cook time: 12 minutes | Serves 4

- 1 pound (454 g) shrimp, shelled and deveined
- ½ cup plain Greek yogurt
- ½ tablespoon chili paste
- ½ tablespoon lime juice
- Chopped green onions, for garnish

Special Equipment:
- Wooden skewers, soaked in water for at least 30 minutes

1. Thread the shrimp onto skewers, piercing once near the tail and once near the head. You can place about 5 shrimps on each skewer.
2. Preheat the grill to medium.
3. Place the shrimp skewers on the grill and cook for about 6 minutes, flipping the shrimp halfway through, or until the shrimp are totally pink and opaque.
4. Meanwhile, make the yogurt and chili sauce: In a small bowl, stir together the yogurt, chili paste, and lime juice.
5. Transfer the shrimp skewers to a large plate. Scatter the green onions on top for garnish and serve with the yogurt and chili sauce on the side.

Per Serving

calories: 122 | fat: 0.8g | protein: 26.1g | carbs: 2.9g | fiber: 0.5g | sugar: 1.3g sodium: 175mg

Mustard Pork Chops

Prep time: 5 minutes | Cook time: 25 minutes | Serves 4

- ¼ cup Dijon mustard
- 1 tablespoon pure maple syrup

From the Cupboard:
- 2 tablespoons rice vinegar
- 4 bone-in, thin-cut pork chops

1. Preheat the oven to 400ºF (205ºC).
2. In a small saucepan, combine the mustard, maple syrup, and rice vinegar. Stir to mix and bring to a simmer over medium heat. Cook for about 2 minutes until just slightly thickened.
3. In a baking dish, place the pork chops and spoon the sauce over them, flipping to coat.
4. Bake, uncovered, for 18 to 22 minutes until the juices run clear.

Per Serving

calories: 258 | fat: 7.1g | protein: 39.1g | carbs: 6.9g | fiber: 0g | sugar: 4.0g sodium: 465mg

Seared Scallops with Orange Sauce

Prep time: 10 minutes | Cook time: 10 minutes | Serves 4

- 2 pounds (907 g) sea scallops, patted dry
- 1 tablespoon minced garlic
- ¼ cup freshly squeezed orange juice

- 1 teaspoon orange zest
- 2 teaspoons chopped fresh thyme, for garnish

From the Cupboard:
- Sea salt and freshly ground black pepper, to taste
- 2 tablespoons extra-virgin olive oil

1. In a bowl, season the scallops with salt and pepper. Set aside.
2. Heat the olive oil in a large skillet over medium-high heat until shimmering.
3. Add the garlic and sauté for about 3 minutes, stirring occasionally, or until the garlic is softened.
4. Add the scallops and cook each side for about 4 minutes, or until the scallops are lightly browned and firm.
5. Remove the scallops from the heat to a plate and cover with foil to keep warm. Set aside.
6. Pour the orange juice and zest into the skillet and stir, scraping up any cooked bits.
7. Drizzle the scallops with the orange sauce and sprinkle the thyme on top for garnish before serving.

Per Serving

calories: 268 | fat: 8.2g | protein: 38.2g | carbs: 8.3g | fiber: 0g | sugar: 1.1g
sodium: 360mg

Grilled Tuna Steaks

Prep time: 5 minutes | Cook time: 10 minutes | Serves 6

- 6 (6-ounce / 170-g) tuna steaks

From the Cupboard:
- 4½ teaspoon olive oil
- ¾ teaspoon salt

- 3 tablespoons fresh basil, diced

- ¼ teaspoon pepper
- Nonstick cooking spray

1. Heat grill to medium heat. Spray rack with cooking spray.
2. Drizzle both sides of the tuna with oil. Sprinkle with basil, salt and pepper.
3. Place on grill and cook 5 minutes per side, tuna should be slightly pink in the center. Serve.

Per Serving

calories: 344 | fat: 14.0g | protein: 51.2g | carbs: 0g | fiber: 0g | sugar: 0g
sodium: 367mg

Salmon Milano

Prep time: 10 minutes | Cook time: 20 minutes | Serves 6

- 2½ pound (1.1 kg) salmon filet
- 2 tomatoes, sliced

From the Cupboard:

- ½ cup margarine

- ½ cup basil pesto

1. Heat the oven to 400ºF (205ºC). Line a baking sheet with foil, making sure it covers the sides. Place another large piece of foil onto the baking sheet and place the salmon filet on top of it.
2. Place the pesto and margarine in blender or food processor and pulse until smooth. Spread evenly over salmon. Place tomato slices on top.
3. Wrap the foil around the salmon, tenting around the top to prevent foil from touching the salmon as much as possible. Bake 15 to 25 minutes, or salmon flakes easily with a fork. Serve.

Per Serving

calories: 445 | fat: 24.0g | protein: 55.2g | carbs: 2.1g | fiber: 0g | sugar: 1.0g sodium: 288mg

Cherry-Glazed Lamb Chops

Prep time: 10 minutes | Cook time: 20 minutes | Serves 4

- 4 (4-ounce / 113-g) lamb chops
- 1½ teaspoons chopped fresh rosemary
- 1 cup frozen cherries, thawed

From the Cupboard:

- ¼ teaspoon salt
- ¼ teaspoon freshly ground black

- ¼ cup dry red wine
- 2 tablespoons orange juice

pepper
- 1 teaspoon extra-virgin olive oil

1. Season the lamb chops with the rosemary, salt, and pepper.
2. In a small saucepan over medium-low heat, combine the cherries, red wine, and orange juice, and simmer, stirring regularly, until the sauce thickens, 8 to 10 minutes.
3. Heat a large skillet over medium-high heat. When the pan is hot, add the olive oil to lightly coat the bottom.
4. Cook the lamb chops for 3 to 4 minutes on each side until well-browned yet medium rare.
5. Serve, topped with the cherry glaze.

Per Serving

calories: 355 | fat: 27.1g | protein: 19.8g | carbs: 5.9g | fiber: 1.0g | sugar: 4.0g sodium: 200mg

Pork Loin, Carrot, and Gold Tomato Roast

- 1 pound (454 g) pork loin
- 2 teaspoons honey
- ½ teaspoon dried rosemary
- 4 (6-inch) carrots, chopped into

½-inch rounds
- 2 small gold potatoes, chopped into 2-inch cubes

From the Cupboard:

- ¼ teaspoon freshly ground black pepper
- 1 tablespoon extra-virgin olive oil, divided

1. Preheat the oven to 350ºF (180ºC).
2. On a clean work surface, rub the pork with honey, rosemary, black pepper, and ½ tablespoon of olive oil. Brush the carrots and gold potatoes with remaining olive oil.
3. Place the pork, carrots, and potatoes in s single layer on a baking sheet.
4. Roast in the preheated oven for 40 minutes or until the pork is lightly browned and the vegetables are soft.
5. Remove them from the oven. Allow to cool for 10 minutes before serving.

Per Serving

calories: 346 | fat: 9.9g | protein: 26.1g | carbs: 25.9g | fiber: 4.1g | sugar: 5.9g sodium: 107mg

Bacon and Cauliflower Casserole

- 6 slices bacon, cooked and crumbled, divided
- 3 scallions, sliced thin, divided
- 5 cup cauliflower
- 2 cup Cheddar cheese, grated and divided
- 1 cup fat free sour cream

From the Cupboard:

- ½ teaspoon salt
- ¼ teaspoon fresh ground black pepper
- Nonstick cooking spray

1. Heat oven to 350ºF (180ºC). Spray casserole dish with cooking spray.
2. Steam cauliflower until just tender.
3. In a large bowl, combine cauliflower, sour cream, half the bacon, half the scallions and half the cheese. Stir in salt and pepper. Place in prepared baking dish and sprinkle remaining cheese over top.
4. Bake 18 to 20 minutes until heated through. Sprinkle remaining scallions and bacon over top and serve.

Per Serving

calories: 333 | fat: 20.0g | protein: 21.1g | carbs: 15.1g | fiber: 4.0g | sugar: 6.0g sodium: 681mg

Roasted Pork Loin with Carrots

Prep time: 5 minutes | Cook time: 40 minutes | Serves 4

- 1 pound (454 g) pork loin
- 2 teaspoons honey
- ½ teaspoon dried rosemary

From the Cupboard:
- 1 tablespoon extra-virgin olive oil, divided

- 4 (6-inch) carrots, chopped into ½-inch rounds

- ¼ teaspoon freshly ground black pepper

1. Preheat the oven to 350ºF (180ºC).
2. Rub the pork loin with ½ tablespoon of oil and the honey. Season with the pepper and rosemary.
3. In a medium bowl, toss the carrots in the remaining ½ tablespoon of oil.
4. Place the pork and the carrots on a baking sheet in a single layer. Cook for 40 minutes.
5. Remove the baking sheet from the oven and let the pork rest for at least 10 minutes before slicing. Divide the pork and carrots into four equal portions.

Per Serving

calories: 344 | fat: 10.1g | protein: 26.1g | carbs: 25.9g | fiber: 3.9g | sugar: 6.0g
sodium: 110mg

Grilled Lamb Racks

Prep time: 15 minutes | Cook time: 20 minutes | Serves 4

- 1 tablespoon garlic, minced
- 2 (1-inch) sprig fresh rosemary
- 2 (1½-pounds / 680-g) French lamb

From the Cupboard:
- 1 tablespoon olive oil, plus more for brushing the grill grates

racks, trimmed of fat, cut into four pieces with two bones, and leave one bone with an equal amount of meat

- ½ teaspoon salt
- Freshly ground black pepper, to taste

1. Combine all the ingredients in a large bowl. Toss to coat the lamb racks well.
2. Wrap the bowl in plastic and refrigerate to marinate for at least 2 hours.
3. Preheat the grill over medium heat. Brush the grill grates with olive oil.
4. Remove the bowl from the refrigerator, and arrange the lamb racks on the grill grates, bone side down.
5. Grill for 3 minutes until lightly browned, then flip the lamb racks, and cover and grill for 15 minutes or until it reaches your desired doneness.
6. Remove the lamb racks from the grill grates and serve hot.

Per Serving

calories: 192 | fat: 9.9g | protein: 22.2g | carbs: 1.0g | fiber: 0g | sugar: 0g
sodium: 347mg

Cod Fillet with Quinoa and Asparagus

Prep time: 5 minutes | Cook time: 15 minutes | Serves 4

- ½ cup uncooked quinoa
- 4 (4-ounce / 113-g) cod fillets
- ½ teaspoon garlic powder, divided

From the Cupboard:

- ¼ teaspoon salt
- ¼ teaspoon freshly ground black

- 24 asparagus spears, cut the bottom 1½ inches off
- 1 cup half-and-half

  pepper
- 1 tablespoon avocado oil

1. Put the quinoa in a pot of salted water. Bring to a boil. Reduce the heat to low and simmer for 15 minutes or until the quinoa is soft and has a white "tail". Cover and turn off the heat. Let sit for 5 minutes.
2. On a clean work surface, rub the cod fillets with ¼ teaspoon of garlic powder, salt, and pepper.
3. Heat the avocado oil in a nonstick skillet over medium-low heat.
4. Add the cod fillets and asparagus in the skillet and cook for 8 minutes or until they are tender. Flip the cod and shake the skillet halfway through the cooking time.
5. Pour the half-and-half in the skillet, and sprinkle with remaining garlic powder. Turn up the heat to high and simmer for 2 minutes until creamy.
6. Divide the quinoa, cod fillets, and asparagus in four bowls and serve warm.

Per Serving

calories: 258 | fat: 7.9g | protein: 25.2g | carbs: 22.7g | fiber: 5.2g | sugar: 3.8g sodium: 410mg

Easy Lime Lamb Cutlets

Prep time: 4 hours 20 minutes | Cook time: 8 minutes | Serves 4

- ¼ cup freshly squeezed lime juice
- 2 tablespoons lime zest
- 2 tablespoons chopped fresh parsley

From the Cupboard:

- Sea salt and freshly ground black pepper, to taste

- 12 lamb cutlets (about 1½ pounds / 680 g in total)

- 1 tablespoon extra-virgin olive oil

1. Combine the lime juice and zest, parsley, salt, black pepper, and olive oil in a large bowl. Stir to mix well.
2. Dunk the lamb cutlets in the bowl of the lime mixture, then toss to coat well. Wrap the bowl in plastic and refrigerate to marinate for at least 4 hours.
3. Preheat the oven to 450ºF (235ºC) or broil. Line a baking sheet with aluminum foil.
4. Remove the bowl from the refrigerator and let sit for 10 minutes, then discard the marinade. Arrange the lamb cutlets on the baking sheet.
5. Broil the lamb in the preheated oven for 8 minutes or until it reaches your desired doneness. Flip the cutlets with tongs to make sure they are cooked evenly.
6. Serve immediately.

Per Serving

calories: 297 | fat: 18.8g | protein: 31.0g | carbs: 1.0g | fiber: 0g | sugar: 0g
sodium: 100mg

CHAPTER 7

SIDE DISH

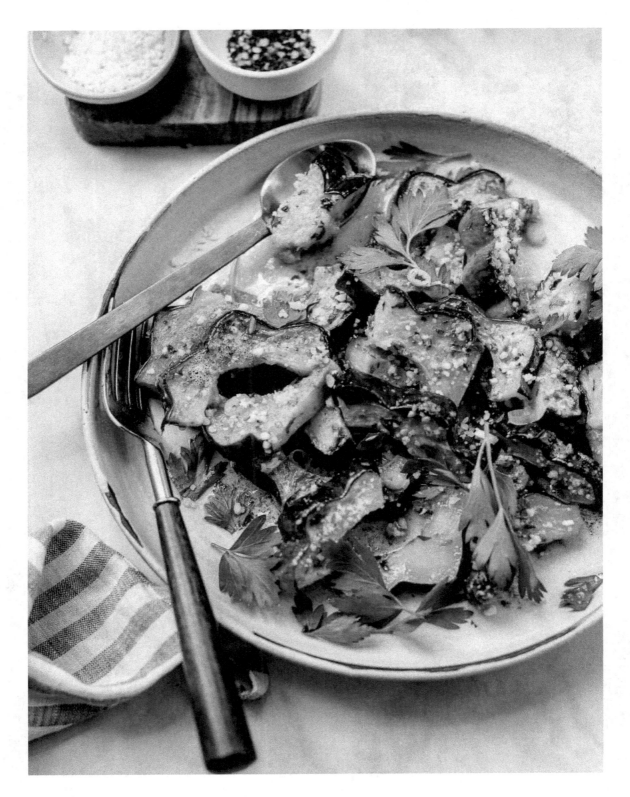

Peppers with Zucchini Dip

Prep time: 10 minutes | Cook time: 0 minutes | Serves 4

- 2 zucchini, chopped
- 3 garlic cloves
- 2 tablespoons tahini

From the Cupboard:

- 2 tablespoons extra-virgin olive oil
- ½ teaspoon sea salt

- Juice of 1 lemon
- 1 red bell pepper, seeded and cut into sticks

1. In a blender or food processor, combine the zucchini, garlic, olive oil, tahini, lemon juice, and salt. Blend until smooth.
2. Serve with the red bell pepper for dipping.

Per Serving

calories: 120 | fat: 11.1g | protein: 2.1g | carbs: 6.9g | fiber: 2.9g | sugar: 4.0g
sodium: 155mg

Simple Parmesan Acorn Squash

Prep time: 10 minutes | Cook time: 20 minutes | Serves 4

- 1 acorn squash (about 1 pound / 454 g)
- 1 teaspoon dried sage leaves, crumbled

From the Cupboard:

- 1 tablespoon extra-virgin olive oil
- ⅛ teaspoon kosher salt

- ¼ teaspoon freshly grated nutmeg
- 2 tablespoons freshly grated Parmesan cheese

- ⅛ teaspoon freshly ground black pepper

1. Cut the acorn squash in half lengthwise and remove the seeds. Cut each half in half for a total of 4 wedges. Snap off the stem if it's easy to do.
2. In a small bowl, combine the olive oil, sage, nutmeg, salt, and pepper. Brush the cut sides of the squash with the olive oil mixture.
3. Pour 1 cup of water into the electric pressure cooker and insert a wire rack or trivet.
4. Place the squash on the trivet in a single layer, skin-side down.
5. Close and lock the lid of the pressure cooker. Set the valve to sealing.
6. Cook on high pressure for 20 minutes.
7. When the cooking is complete, hit Cancel and quick release the pressure.
8. Once the pin drops, unlock and remove the lid.
9. Carefully remove the squash from the pot, sprinkle with the Parmesan, and serve.

Per Serving

calories: 86 | fat: 4.1g | protein: 2.1g | carbs: 11.9g | fiber: 2.1g | sugar: 0g
sodium: 283mg

Hearty Corn on the Cob

Prep time: 10 minutes | Cook time: 20 minutes | Serves 12

- 6 ears corn

1. Remove the husks and silk from the corn. Cut or break each ear in half.
2. Pour 1 cup of water into the bottom of the electric pressure cooker. Insert a wire rack or trivet.
3. Place the corn upright on the rack, cut-side down. Close and lock the lid of the pressure cooker. Set the valve to sealing.
4. Cook on high pressure for 5 minutes.
5. When the cooking is complete, hit Cancel and quick release the pressure.
6. Once the pin drops, unlock and remove the lid.
7. Use tongs to remove the corn from the pot. Season as desired and serve immediately.

Per Serving

calories: 64 | fat: 1.1g | protein: 2.1g | carbs: 13.9g | fiber: 0.9g | sugar: 5.0g
sodium: 12mg

Roasted Cauliflower with Lime Juice

Prep time: 5 minutes | Cook time: 25 minutes | Serves 4

- 1 cauliflower head, broken into small florets
- ½ teaspoon ground chipotle chili powder
- Juice of 1 lime

From the Cupboard:
- 2 tablespoons extra-virgin olive oil
- ½ teaspoon salt, or more to taste

1. Preheat the oven to 450ºF (235ºC) and line a large baking sheet with parchment paper. Set aside.
2. Toss the cauliflower florets in the olive oil in a large bowl. Season with salt and chipotle chili powder.
3. Arrange the cauliflower florets on the baking sheet.
4. Roast in the preheated oven for 15 minutes until lightly browned. Flip the cauliflower and continue to roast until crisp and tender, about 10 minutes.
5. Remove from the oven and season as needed with salt.
6. Cool for 6 minutes and drizzle with the lime juice, then serve.

Per Serving

calories: 100 | fat: 7.1g | protein: 3.2g | carbs: 8.1g | fiber: 3.2g | sugar: 3.2g
sodium: 285mg

Vegetable Stuffed Portobello Mushrooms

Prep time: 5 minutes | Cook time: 20 minutes | Serves 4

- 8 large portobello mushrooms
- 4 cups fresh spinach

From the Cupboard:
- 3 teaspoons extra-virgin olive oil, divided

- 1 medium red bell pepper, diced
- ¼ cup feta cheese, crumbled

1. Preheat the oven to 450ºF (235ºC).
2. On your cutting board, remove the mushroom stems. Scoop out the gills with a spoon and discard. Grease the mushrooms with 2 tablespoons olive oil.
3. Arrange the mushrooms, cap-side down, on a baking sheet. Roast in the preheated oven for 20 minutes until browned on top.
4. Meanwhile, in a skillet, heat the remaining olive oil over medium heat until shimmering.
5. Add the spinach and red bell pepper to the skillet and sauté for 8 minutes until the vegetables are tender, stirring occasionally. Remove from the heat to a bowl.
6. Remove the mushrooms from the oven to a plate. Using a spoon to stuff the mushrooms with the vegetables and sprinkle with the feta cheese. Serve warm.

Per Serving

calories: 118 | fat: 6.3g | protein: 7.2g | carbs: 12.2g | fiber: 4.1g | sugar: 6.1g
sodium: 128mg

Sauteed Green Beans with Nutmeg

Prep time: 15 minutes | Cook time: 5 minutes | Serves 4

- 1½ pounds (680 g) green beans, trimmed

From the Cupboard:
- 1 tablespoon butter

- 1 teaspoon ground nutmeg

- Sea salt, to taste

1. Melt the butter in a large skillet over medium heat.
2. Sauté the green beans in the melted butter for 5 minutes until tender but still crisp, stirring frequently.
3. Season with nutmeg and salt and mix well.
4. Remove from the heat and cool for a few minutes before serving.

Per Serving

calories: 83 | fat: 3.2g | protein: 3.2g | carbs: 12.2g | fiber: 6.1g | sugar: 3.2g
sodium: 90mg

Sautéed Collard Greens and Cabbage

Prep time: 10 minutes | Cook time: 10 minutes | Serves 8

- 1 collard greens bunch, stemmed and thinly sliced

From the Cupboard:
- 2 tablespoons extra-virgin olive oil

- ½ small green cabbage, thinly sliced
- 6 garlic cloves, minced

- 1 tablespoon low-sodium soy sauce

1. Heat the olive oil in a large skillet over medium-high heat.
2. Sauté the collard greens in the oil for about 2 minutes, or until the greens start to wilt.
3. Toss in the cabbage and mix well. Reduce the heat to medium-low, cover, and cook for 5 to 7 minutes, stirring occasionally, or until the greens are softened.
4. Fold in the garlic and soy sauce and stir to combine. Cook for about 30 seconds more until fragrant.
5. Remove from the heat to a plate and serve.

Per Serving

calories: 73 | fat: 4.1g | protein: 3.2g | carbs: 5.9g | fiber: 2.9g | sugar: 0g
sodium: 128mg

Roasted Delicata Squash with Thyme

Prep time: 10 minutes | Cook time: 20 minutes | Serves 4

- 1 (1- to 1½-pound) delicata squash, halved, seeded, and cut into ½-inch-thick strips
- ½ teaspoon dried thyme

From the Cupboard:
- 1 tablespoon extra-virgin olive oil
- ¼ teaspoon salt

- ¼ teaspoon freshly ground black pepper

1. Preheat the oven to 400ºF (205ºC). Line a baking sheet with parchment paper and set aside.
2. Add the squash strips, olive oil, thyme, salt, and pepper in a large bowl, and toss until the squash strips are fully coated.
3. Place the squash strips on the prepared baking sheet in a single layer. Roast for about 20 minutes until lightly browned, flipping the strips halfway through.
4. Remove from the oven and serve on plates.

Per Serving

calories: 78 | fat: 4.2g | protein: 1.1g | carbs: 11.8g | fiber: 2.1g | sugar: 2.9g
sodium: 122mg

Roasted Asparagus and Red Peppers

Prep time: 5 minutes | Cook time: 15 minutes | Serves 4

- 1 pound (454 g) asparagus, woody ends trimmed, cut into 2-inch segments
- 2 red bell peppers, seeded, cut into 1-inch pieces
- 1 small onion, quartered
- 2 tablespoons Italian dressing

1. Preheat the oven to 400ºF (205ºC). Line a baking sheet with parchment paper and set aside.
2. Combine the asparagus with the peppers, onion, and dressing in a large bowl, and toss well.
3. Arrange the vegetables on the baking sheet and roast for about 15 minutes until softened. Flip the vegetables with a spatula once during cooking.
4. Transfer to a large platter and serve.

Per Serving

calories: 92 | fat: 4.8g | protein: 2.9g | carbs: 10.7g | fiber: 4.0g | sugar: 5.7g
sodium: 31mg

Garlicky Broccoli Florets

Prep time: 10 minutes | Cook time: 25 minutes | Serves 8

- 2 large broccoli heads, cut into florets
- 3 garlic cloves, minced

From the Cupboard:
- 2 tablespoons extra-virgin olive oil
- ¼ teaspoon salt
- 2 tablespoons freshly squeezed lemon juice
- ¼ teaspoon ground black pepper

1. Preheat the oven to 425ºF (220ºC) and line a large baking sheet with parchment paper.
2. In a large bowl, add the broccoli, olive oil, garlic, salt, and pepper. Toss well until the broccoli is coated completely. Transfer the broccoli to the prepared baking sheet.
3. Roast in the preheated oven for about 25 minutes, flipping the broccoli halfway through, or until the broccoli is browned and fork-tender.
4. Remove from the oven to a plate and let cool for 5 minutes. Serve drizzled with the lemon juice.

Per Serving

calories: 33 | fat: 2.1g | protein: 1.2g | carbs: 3.1g | fiber: 1.1g | sugar: 1.1g
sodium: 85mg

Tarragon Spring Peas

Prep time: 10 minutes | Cook time: 12 minutes | Serves 6 (½ cup each)

- ½ Vidalia onion, thinly sliced
- 1 cup low-sodium vegetable broth

From the Cupboard:

- 1 tablespoon unsalted butter

- 3 cups fresh shelled peas
- 1 tablespoon minced fresh tarragon

1. Melt the butter in a skillet over medium heat.
2. Sauté the onion in the melted butter for about 3 minutes until translucent, stirring occasionally.
3. Pour in the vegetable broth and whisk well. Add the peas and tarragon to the skillet and stir to combine.
4. Reduce the heat to low, cover, and cook for about 8 minutes more, or until the peas are tender.
5. Let the peas cool for 5 minutes and serve warm.

Per Serving

calories: 82 | fat: 2.1g | protein: 4.2g | carbs: 12.0g | fiber: 3.8g | sugar: 4.9g
sodium: 48mg

Roasted Tomato Brussels Sprouts

Prep time: 15 minutes | Cook time: 20 minutes | Serves 4

- 1 pound (454 g) Brussels sprouts, trimmed and halved
- ½ cup sun-dried tomatoes, chopped

From the Cupboard:

- 1 tablespoon extra-virgin olive oil
- Sea salt and freshly ground black pepper, to taste

- 2 tablespoons freshly squeezed lemon juice
- 1 teaspoon lemon zest

1. Preheat the oven to 400ºF (205ºC). Line a large baking sheet with aluminum foil.
2. Toss the Brussels sprouts in the olive oil in a large bowl until well coated. Sprinkle with salt and pepper.
3. Spread out the seasoned Brussels sprouts on the prepared baking sheet in a single layer.
4. Roast in the preheated oven for 20 minutes, shaking the pan halfway through, or until the Brussels sprouts are crispy and browned on the outside.
5. Remove from the oven to a serving bowl. Add the tomatoes, lemon juice, and lemon zest, and stir to incorporate. Serve immediately.

Per Serving

calories: 111 | fat: 5.8g | protein: 5.0g | carbs: 13.7g | fiber: 4.9g | sugar: 2.7g
sodium: 103mg

Simple Sautéed Greens

Prep time: 10 minutes | Cook time: 10 minutes | Serves 4

- 1 pound (454 g) Swiss chard, coarse stems removed and leaves chopped
- 1 pound (454 g) kale, coarse stems removed and leaves chopped

From the Cupboard:
- 2 tablespoons extra-virgin olive oil

- ½ teaspoon ground cardamom
- 1 tablespoon freshly squeezed lemon juice

- Sea salt and freshly ground black pepper, to taste

1. Heat the olive oil in a large skillet over medium-high heat.
2. Add the Swiss chard, kale, cardamon, and lemon juice to the skillet, and stir to combine. Cook for about 10 minutes, stirring continuously, or until the greens are wilted.
3. Sprinkle with the salt and pepper and stir well.
4. Serve the greens on a plate while warm.

Per Serving

calories: 139 | fat: 6.8g | protein: 5.9g | carbs: 15.8g | fiber: 3.9g | sugar: 1.0g
sodium: 350mg

Garlicky Mushrooms

Prep time: 10 minutes | Cook time: 12 minutes | Serves 4

- 2 pounds (907 g) button mushrooms, halved

From the Cupboard:
- 1 tablespoon butter
- 2 teaspoons extra-virgin olive oil

- 2 teaspoons minced fresh garlic
- 1 teaspoon chopped fresh thyme

- Sea salt and freshly ground black pepper, to taste

1. Heat the butter and olive oil in a large skillet over medium-high heat.
2. Add the mushrooms and sauté for 10 minutes, stirring occasionally, or until the mushrooms are lightly browned and cooked though.
3. Stir in the garlic and thyme and cook for an additional 2 minutes.
4. Season with salt and pepper and serve on a plate.

Per Serving

calories: 96 | fat: 6.1g | protein: 6.9g | carbs: 8.2g | fiber: 1.7g | sugar: 3.9g
sodium: 91mg

Lemony Brussels Sprouts

Prep time: 10 minutes | Cook time: 20 minutes | Serves 4

- 1 pound (454 g) Brussels sprouts
- 1 cup vegetable broth or chicken bone broth

From the Cupboard:
- 2 tablespoons avocado oil, divided
- ½ teaspoon kosher salt

- 1 tablespoon minced garlic
- ½ medium lemon
- ½ tablespoon poppy seeds

- Freshly ground black pepper, to taste

1. Trim the Brussels sprouts by cutting off the stem ends and removing any loose outer leaves. Cut each in half lengthwise (through the stem).
2. Set the electric pressure cooker to the Sauté/More setting. When the pot is hot, pour in 1 tablespoon of the avocado oil.
3. Add half of the Brussels sprouts to the pot, cut-side down, and let them brown for 3 to 5 minutes without disturbing. Transfer to a bowl and add the remaining tablespoon of avocado oil and the remaining Brussels sprouts to the pot. Hit Cancel and return all of the Brussels sprouts to the pot.
4. Add the broth, garlic, salt, and a few grinds of pepper. Stir to distribute the seasonings.
5. Close and lock the lid of the pressure cooker. Set the valve to sealing.
6. Cook on high pressure for 2 minutes.
7. While the Brussels sprouts are cooking, zest the lemon, then cut it into quarters.
8. When the cooking is complete, hit Cancel and quick release the pressure.
9. Once the pin drops, unlock and remove the lid.
10. Using a slotted spoon, transfer the Brussels sprouts to a serving bowl. Toss with the lemon zest, a squeeze of lemon juice, and the poppy seeds. Serve immediately.

Per Serving

calories: 126 | fat: 8.1g | protein: 4.1g | carbs: 12.9g | fiber: 4.9g | sugar: 3.0g
sodium: 500mg

CHAPTER 8

SNACK

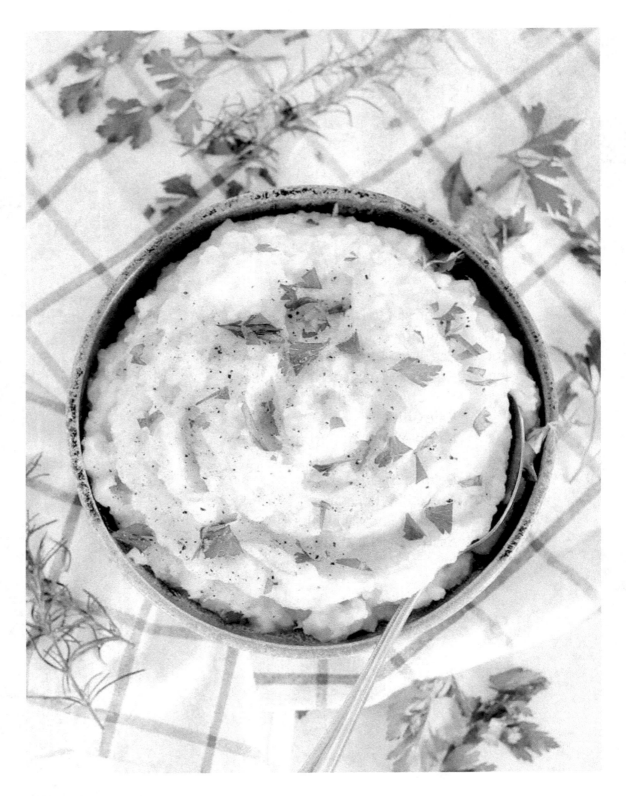

Parmesan Crisps

- 1 cup grated Parmesan cheese

1. Preheat the oven to 400ºF (205ºC). Line a rimmed baking sheet with parchment paper.
2. Spread the Parmesan on the prepared baking sheet into 4 mounds, spreading each mound out so it is flat but not touching the others.
3. Bake until brown and crisp, 3 to 5 minutes.
4. Cool for 5 minutes. Use a spatula to remove to a plate to continue cooling.

Per Serving

calories: 216 | fat: 14.1g | protein: 19.1g | carbs: 2.0g | fiber: 0g | sugar: 1.5g
sodium: 765mg

Cauliflower Mash

- 1 head cauliflower, cored and cut into large florets
- ½ teaspoon garlic pepper
- 2 tablespoons plain Greek yogurt
- ¾ cup freshly grated Parmesan cheese
- Chopped fresh chives

From the Cupboard:
- ½ teaspoon kosher salt
- 1 tablespoon unsalted butter or ghee (optional)

1. Pour 1 cup of water into the electric pressure cooker and insert a steamer basket or wire rack.
2. Place the cauliflower in the basket.
3. Close and lock the lid of the pressure cooker. Set the valve to sealing.
4. Cook on high pressure for 5 minutes.
5. When the cooking is complete, hit Cancel and quick release the pressure.
6. Once the pin drops, unlock and remove the lid.
7. Remove the cauliflower from the pot and pour out the water. Return the cauliflower to the pot and add the salt, garlic pepper, yogurt, and cheese. Use an immersion blender or potato masher to purée or mash the cauliflower in the pot.
8. Spoon into a serving bowl, and garnish with butter (if using) and chives.

Per Serving

calories: 141 | fat: 6.1g | protein: 12.1g | carbs: 11.9g | fiber: 4.1g | sugar: 5.0g
sodium: 591mg

Easy Low-Carb Biscuits

Prep time: 10 minutes | Cook time: 15 minutes | Serves 4 biscuits

- ¼ cup plain Greek yogurt
- 1½ cups finely ground almond flour

From the Cupboard:

- 2 tablespoons unsalted butter, melted
- Pinch salt

1. Preheat the oven to 375ºF (190ºC).
2. Combine the yogurt, butter, and salt in a bowl. Stir to mix well.
3. Fold the almond flour in the mixture. Keep stirring until a dough without lumps forms.
4. Divide the dough into 4 balls, then bash the balls into 1-inch biscuits with your hands.
5. Arrange the biscuits on a baking pan lined with parchment paper. Bake in the preheated oven for 14 minutes or until well browned.
6. Remove the biscuits from the oven and serve warm.

Per Serving

calories: 312 | fat: 27.9g | protein: 10.2g | carbs: 8.9g | fiber: 5.1g | sugar: 2.1g
sodium: 31mg

Aromatic Toasted Pumpkin Seeds

Prep time: 5 minutes | Cook time: 45 minutes | Serves 4

- 1 cup pumpkin seeds
- 1 teaspoon cinnamon
- 2 (0.04-ounce / 1-g) packets stevia

From the Cupboard:

- 1 tablespoon canola oil
- ¼ teaspoon sea salt

1. Preheat the oven to 300°F (150°C).
2. Combine the pumpkin seeds with cinnamon, stevia, canola oil and salt in a bowl. Stir to mix well.
3. Pour the seeds in the single layer on a baking sheet, then arrange the sheet in the preheated oven.
4. Bake for 45 minutes or until well toasted and fragrant. Shake the sheet twice to bake the seeds evenly.
5. Serve immediately.

Per Serving

calories: 202 | fat: 18.0g | protein: 8.8g | carbs: 5.1g | fiber: 2.3g | sugar: 0.4g
sodium: 151mg

Hot Chicken Stuffed Celery Stalks

Prep time: 10 minutes | Cook time: 0 minutes | Serves 4

- 1 teaspoon Buffalo hot sauce
- ¼ cup chunky blue cheese dressing
- 1 cup rotisserie chicken meat, shredded
- 8 celery stalks, cut into halves lengthwise

1. Combine the hot sauce and blue cheese dressing in a bowl, then dunk the shredded rotisserie chicken in the bowl to coat well.
2. Divide the mixture in the celery stalks and serve.

Per Serving

calories: 148 | fat: 11.9g | protein: 9.1g | carbs: 2.8g | fiber: 1.2g | carbs: 1.6g
sodium: 461mg

Kale Chips

Prep time: 5 minutes | Cook time: 15 minutes | Serves 1

- ¼ teaspoon garlic powder
- 1 (8-ounce / 227-g) bunch kale, trimmed and cut into 2-inch pieces, rinsed

From the Cupboard:

- Pinch cayenne, to taste
- 1 tablespoon extra-virgin olive oil
- ½ teaspoon sea salt, or to taste

1. Preheat the oven to 350ºF (180ºC). Line two baking sheets with parchment paper.
2. Combine the garlic powder, cayenne pepper, olive oil, and salt in a large bowl, then dunk the kale in the bowl. Toss to coat well.
3. Place the kale in the single layer on one of the baking sheet.
4. Arrange the sheet in the preheated oven and bake for 7 minutes. Remove the sheet from the oven and pour the kale in the single layer of the other baking sheet.
5. Move the sheet of kale back to the oven and bake for another 7 minutes or until the kale is crispy.
6. Serve immediately.

Per Serving

calories: 136 | fat: 14.0g | protein: 1.0g | carbs: 3.0g | fiber: 1.1g | sugar: 0.6g
sodium: 1170mg

Bacon-Wrapped Shrimps

Prep time: 10 minutes | Cook time: 6 minutes | Serves 10

- 20 shrimps, peeled and deveined
- 7 slices bacon, cut into 3 strips
- crosswise
- 4 leaves romaine lettuce

1. Preheat the oven to 400ºF (205ºC).
2. Wrap each shrimp with each bacon strip, then arrange the wrapped shrimps in a single layer on a baking sheet, seam side down.
3. Broil in the preheated oven for 6 minutes or until the bacon is well browned. Flip the shrimps halfway through the cooking time.
4. Remove the shrimps from the oven and serve on lettuce leaves.

Per Serving

calories: 70 | fat: 4.5g | protein: 7.0g | carbs: 0g | fiber: 0g | sugar: 0g
sodium: 150mg

Caprese Skewers

Prep time: 5 minutes | Cook time: 0 minutes | Serves 2

- 12 cherry tomatoes
- 8 (1-inch) pieces Mozzarella cheese
- 12 basil leaves
- ¼ cup Italian vinaigrette, for serving

Special Equipment:
- 4 wooden skewers, soaked in water for at least 30 minutes

1. Thread the tomatoes, cheese, and bay leaves alternatively through the skewers.
2. Place the skewers on a large plate and baste with the Italian Vinaigrette. Serve immediately.

Per Serving

calories: 230 | fat: 12.6g | protein: 21.3g | carbs: 8.5g | fiber: 1.9g | sugar: 4.9g
sodium: 672mg

Deviled Eggs

Prep time: 5 minutes | Cook time: 8 minutes | Serves 12

- 6 large eggs
- ⅛ teaspoon mustard powder
- 2 tablespoons plus 1 teaspoon light mayonnaise

From the Cupboard:
- Salt and freshly ground black pepper, to taste

1. Sit the eggs in a saucepan, then pour in enough water to cover the egg. Bring to a boil, then boil the eggs for another 8 minutes. Turn off the heat and cover, then let sit for 15 minutes.
2. Transfer the boiled eggs in a pot of cold water and peel under the water.
3. Transfer the eggs on a large plate, then cut in half. Remove the egg yolks and place them in a bowl, then mash with a fork.
4. Add the mustard powder, mayo, salt, and pepper to the bowl of yolks, then stir to mix well.
5. Spoon the yolk mixture in the egg white on the plate. Serve immediately.

Per Serving

calories: 45 | fat: 3.0g | protein: 3.0g | carbs: 1.0g | fiber: 0g | sugar: 0g
sodium: 70mg

Apple Pita Pockets

Prep time: 10 minutes | Cook time: 2 minutes | Serves 2

- ½ apple, cored and chopped
- ½ teaspoon cinnamon
- ¼ cup almond butter
- 1 whole-wheat pita, halved

1. Combine the apple, cinnamon, and almond butter in a bowl. Stir to mix well.
2. Heat the pita in a nonstick skillet over medium heat until lightly browned on both sides.
3. Remove the pita from the skillet. Allow to cool for a few minutes. Spoon the mixture in the halved pita pockets, then serve.

Per Serving

calories: 315 | fat: 20.3g | protein: 8.2g | carbs: 31.3g | fiber: 7.2g | sugar: 20.6g
sodium: 175mg

Almond Cheesecake Bites

Prep time: 5 minutes | Cook time: 0 minutes | Serves 6

- ½ cup reduced-fat cream cheese, soft
- ½ cup ground almonds
- ¼ cup almond butter
- 2 drops liquid stevia

1. In a large bowl, beat cream cheese, almond butter and stevia on high speed until mixture is smooth and creamy. Cover and chill 30 minutes.
2. Use your hands to shape the mixture into 12 balls.
3. Place the ground almonds in a shallow plate. Roll the balls in the nuts completely covering all sides. Store in an airtight container in the refrigerator.

Per Serving

calories: 70 | fat: 4.9g | protein: 5.1g | carbs: 3.1g | fiber: 1g | sugar: 0g
sodium: 73mg

Asian Chicken Wings

Prep time: 5 minutes | Cook time: 30 minutes | Serves 3

- 24 chicken wings
From the Cupboard:
- 6 tablespoons soy sauce
- Salt and ground black pepper, to taste
- 6 tablespoons Chinese 5 spice
- Nonstick cooking spray

1. Heat oven to 350ºF (180ºC). Spray a baking sheet with cooking spray.
2. Combine the soy sauce, 5 spice, salt, and pepper in a large bowl. Add the wings and toss to coat.
3. Pour the wings onto the prepared pan. Bake for 15 minutes. Turn chicken over and cook another 15 minutes until chicken is cooked through.
4. Serve warm.

Per Serving

calories: 180 | fat: 10.9g | protein: 12.1g | carbs: 8.1g | fiber: 0g | sugar: 1.0g
sodium: 1210mg

CHAPTER 9

DESSERT

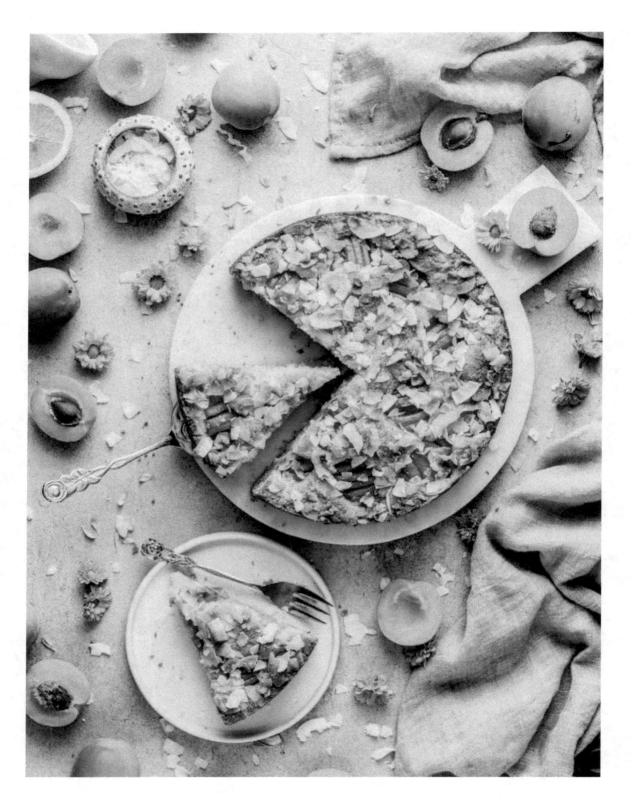

Orange and Peach Ambrosia

Prep time: 10 minutes | Cook time: 0 minutes | Serves 8

- 3 oranges, peeled, sectioned, and quartered
- 2 (4-ounce / 113-g) cups diced peaches in water, drained
- 1 cup shredded, unsweetened coconut
- 1 (8-ounce / 227-g) container fat-free crème fraîche

1. In a large mixing bowl, combine the oranges, peaches, coconut, and crème fraîche. Gently toss until well mixed. Cover and refrigerate overnight.

Per Serving

calories: 113 | fat: 5.1g | protein: 2.1g | carbs: 12.1g | fiber: 2.9g | sugar: 8.1g
sodium: 8mg

Coconut Milk Shakes

Prep time: 5 minutes | Cook time: 0 minutes | Serves 2

- 1½ cup vanilla ice cream
- ½ cup coconut milk, unsweetened
- 2½ tablespoons coconut flakes
- 1 teaspoon unsweetened cocoa

1. Heat oven to 350ºF (180ºC).
2. Place coconut on a baking sheet and bake, 2 to 3 minutes, stirring often, until coconut is toasted.
3. Place ice cream, milk, 2 tablespoons coconut, and cocoa in a blender and process until smooth.
4. Pour into glasses and garnish with remaining toasted coconut. Serve immediately.

Per Serving

calories: 324 | fat: 24.0g | protein: 3.0g | carbs: 23.1g | fiber: 4.0g | sugar: 18.1g
sodium: 107mg

Coconut Yogurt and Pistachio Stuffed Peaches

Prep time: 5 minutes | Cook time: 10 minutes | Serves 4

- 2 peaches, halved and pitted
- 1 teaspoon pure vanilla extract
- ½ cup plain Greek yogurt
- 2 tablespoons unsalted pistachios,
- shelled and broken into pieces
- ¼ cup unsweetened dried coconut flakes

1. Preheat the broiler to high.
2. Place the peach halves on a baking sheet, cut side down, and broil for 7 minutes or until soft and lightly browned.

3. Meanwhile, combine the vanilla and yogurt in a bowl.
4. Divide the mixture among the the pits of peach halves, then scatter the pistachios and coconut flakes on top before serving.

Per Serving

calories: 103 | fat: 4.9g | protein: 5.1g | carbs: 10.8g | fiber: 2.1g | sugars: 7.8g sodium: 10mg

Strawberry and Rhubarb Glazed Ice Cream

Prep time: 10 minutes | Cook time: 15 minutes | Serves 4

- 1 cup strawberries, sliced
- 1 cup rhubarb, chopped
- 1 tablespoon honey

From the Cupboard:
- 2 tablespoons water

- ½ teaspoon cinnamon
- ¼ cup sugar-free vanilla ice cream

1. Combine all the ingredients, except for the ice cream, in a pot.
2. Bring to a boil over medium heat, then turn down the heat to medium-low. Simmer for 15 minutes or until the rhubarb is tender. Stir constantly.
3. Divide the ice cream on four small plates with a spoon, then pour the mixture over the ice cream before serving.

Per Serving

calories: 88 | fat: 2.1g | protein: 3.1g | carbs: 15.8g | fiber: 3.2g | carbs: 12.6g sodium: 35mg

Crispy Apple and Pecan Bake

Prep time: 10 minutes | Cook time: 15 minutes | Serves 4

- 2 apples, peeled, cored, and chopped
- ½ teaspoon cinnamon
- ½ teaspoon ground ginger

- 2 tablespoons pure maple syrup
- ¼ cup pecans, chopped

1. Preheat the oven to 350ºF (180ºC).
2. Combine all the ingredients, except for the pecans, in a bowl. Stir to mix well.
3. Pour the mixture in a baking dish, and spread the pecans over the mixture.
4. Bake in the preheated oven for 15 minutes or until the apples are soft.
5. Remove them from the oven and serve warm.

Per Serving

calories: 124 | fat: 5.1g | protein: 1.1g | carbs: 20.8g | fiber: 3.2g | carbs: 18.6g sodium: 1mg

Apple Cinnamon Chimichanga

Prep time: 15 minutes | Cook time: 15 minutes | Serves 4

- 2 apple, cored and chopped
- 3 tablespoons Splenda, divided

From the Cupboard:
- ¼ cup water

- ½ teaspoon ground cinnamon
- 4 (8-inch) whole-wheat flour tortillas

- Nonstick cooking spray

Special Equipment:
- 4 toothpicks, soaked in water for at least 30 minutes

1. Preheat the oven to 400ºF (205ºC). Line a baking sheet with parchment paper and set aside.
2. Make the apple filling: Add the apples, 2 tablespoons of Splenda, water, and cinnamon to a medium saucepan over medium heat. Stir to combine and allow the mixture to boil for 5 minutes, or until the apples are fork-tender, but not mushy.
3. Remove the apple filling from the heat and let it cool to room temperature.
4. Make the chimichangas: Place the tortillas on a lightly floured surface.
5. Spoon 2 teaspoons of prepared apple filling onto each tortilla and fold the tortilla over to enclose the filling. Roll each tortilla up and run the toothpicks through to secure. Spritz the tortillas lightly with nonstick cooking spray.
6. Arrange the tortillas on the prepared baking sheet, seam-side down. Scatter the remaining Splenda all over the tortillas.
7. Bake in the preheated oven for 10 minutes, flipping the tortillas halfway through, or until they are crispy and golden brown on each side.
8. Remove from the oven to four plates and serve while warm.

Per Serving (1 Chimichanga)
calories: 201 | fat: 6.2g | protein: 3.9g | carbs: 32.8g | fiber: 5.0g | sugar: 7.9g
sodium: 241mg

Peanut Butter and Pineapple Smoothie

Prep time: 10 minutes | Cook time: 0 minutes | Serves 6

- 1 cup peanut butter
- 2 cups frozen pineapple

- ½ cup unsweetened almond milk

1. Put the peanut butter and pineapple in a food processor, then pour the almond milk in the food processor.
2. Pulse until creamy and smooth, then pour the mixture into 6 glasses and serve.

Per Serving
calories: 303 | fat: 21.8g | protein: 14.1g | carbs: 14.8g | fiber: 4.2g | sugars: 7.8g
sodium: 37mg

Apple Chips

Prep time: 10 minutes | Cook time: 2 hours | Serves 4

- 2 medium apples, sliced
- 1 teaspoon ground cinnamon

1. Preheat the oven to 200ºF (93ºC). Line a baking sheet with parchment paper.
2. Arrange the apple slices on the prepared baking sheet, then sprinkle with cinnamon.
3. Bake in the preheated oven for 2 hours or until crispy. Flip the apple chips halfway through the cooking time.
4. Allow to cool for 10 minutes and serve warm.

Per Serving

calories: 50 | fat: 0g | protein: 0g | carbs: 13.0g | fiber: 2.0g | sugar: 9.0g
sodium: 0mg

Blackberry Crostata

Prep time: 10 minutes | Cook time: 20 minutes | Serves 6

- 1 (9-inch) pie crust, unbaked
- 2 cup fresh blackberries
- Juice and zest of 1 lemon
- 3 tablespoons Splenda, divided
- 2 tablespoons cornstarch

From the Cupboard:
- 2 tablespoons butter, soft

1. Heat oven to 425ºF (220ºC). Line a large baking sheet with parchment paper and unroll pie crust in pan.
2. In a medium bowl, combine blackberries, 2 tablespoons Splenda, lemon juice and zest, and cornstarch. Spoon onto crust leaving a 2-inch edge. Fold and crimp the edges.
3. Dot the berries with 1 tablespoon butter. Brush the crust edge with remaining butter and sprinkle crust and fruit with remaining Splenda.
4. Bake for 20 to 22 minutes or until golden brown. Cool before cutting and serving.

Per Serving

calories: 207 | fat: 11.1g | protein: 2.0g | carbs: 24.1g | fiber: 3.0g | sugar: 9.1g
sodium: 226mg

Blackberry Soufflés

Prep time: 15 minutes | Cook time: 30 minutes | Serves 4

- 12 ounces (340 g) blackberries
- 4 egg whites

From the Cupboard:
- 1 tablespoon water

- ⅓ cup Splenda
- 1 tablespoon Swerve powdered sugar

- Nonstick cooking spray

1. Heat oven to 375ºF (190ºC). Spray 4 1-cup ramekins with cooking spray.
2. In a small saucepan, over medium-high heat, combine blackberries and 1 tablespoon water, bring to a boil. Reduce heat and simmer until berries are soft. Add Splenda and stir over medium heat until Splenda dissolves, without boiling.
3. Bring back to boiling, reduce heat and simmer 5 minutes. Remove from heat and cool 5 minutes.
4. Place a fine meshed sieve over a small bowl and push the berry mixture through it using the back of a spoon. Discard the seeds. Cover and chill 15 minutes.
5. In a large bowl, beat egg whites until soft peaks form. Gently fold in berry mixture. Spoon evenly into prepared ramekins and place them on a baking sheet.
6. Bake 12 minutes, or until puffed and light brown. Dust with powdered Swerve and serve immediately.

Per Serving

calories: 142 | fat: 0g | protein: 5.0g | carbs: 26.1g | fiber: 5.0g | sugar: 20.1g
sodium: 56mg

Avocado Mousse with Grilled Watermelon

Prep time: 10 minutes | Cook time: 10 minutes | Serves 8

- 1 small, seedless watermelon, halved and cut into 1-inch rounds

From the Cupboard:
- ¼ teaspoon cayenne pepper

- 2 ripe avocados, pitted and peeled
- ½ cup fat-free plain yogurt

1. On a hot grill, grill the watermelon slices for 2 to 3 minutes on each side, or until you can see the grill marks.
2. To make the avocado mousse, in a blender, combine the avocados, yogurt, and cayenne and process until smooth.
3. To serve, cut each watermelon round in half. Top each with a generous dollop of avocado mousse.

Per Serving

calories: 127 | fat: 3.9g | protein: 3.1g | carbs: 24.1g | fiber: 2.9g | sugar: 16.9g
sodium: 15mg

Baked Maple Custard

Prep time: 5 minutes | Cook time: 1 hour 15 minutes | Serves 6

- 2½ cup half-and-half
- ½ cup egg substitute
- ¼ cup Splenda

From the Cupboard:

- 3 cup boiling water

- 2 tablespoons sugar free maple syrup
- 2 teaspoons vanilla

- Nonstick cooking spray

1. Heat oven to 325ºF (163ºC). Lightly spray 6 custard cups or ramekins with cooking spray.
2. In a large bowl, whisk together half-and-half, egg substitute, Splenda, and vanilla. Pour evenly into prepared custard cups. Place cups in a baking dish.
3. Pour boiling water around, being careful not to splash it into, the cups. Bake 1 hour 15 minutes, centers will not be completely set.
4. Remove cups from pan and cool completely. Cover and chill overnight.
5. Just before serving, drizzle with the maple syrup.

Per Serving

calories: 191 | fat: 12.1g | protein: 5.0g | carbs: 15.1g | fiber: 0g | sugar: 8.1g
sodium: 152mg

Broiled Stone Fruit

Prep time: 5 minutes | Cook time: 5 minutes | Serves 2

- 1 peach
- 1 nectarine
- 2 tablespoons sugar free whipped topping

- 1 tablespoon Splenda brown sugar
- From the Cupboard:
- Nonstick cooking spray

1. Heat oven to broil. Line a shallow baking dish with foil and spray with cooking spray.
2. Cut the peach and nectarine in half and remove pits. Place cut side down in prepared dish. Broil 3 minutes.
3. Turn fruit over and sprinkle with Splenda brown sugar. Broil another 2 to 3 minutes.
4. Transfer 1 of each fruit to a dessert bowl and top with 1 tablespoon of whipped topping. Serve.

Per Serving

calories: 100 | fat: 1.0g | protein: 1.0g | carbs: 22.1g | fiber: 2.0g | sugar: 19.1g
sodium: 0mg

CONCLUSION

I hope you have enjoyed these recipes as much as I have. Life with diabetes should not be hard. It is not the end—it is the beginning. With healthy dietary management, you can lead a life free from the negative effects of high (or low) blood sugar levels. With the knowledge I have shared, you now know why you may have become diabetic, you know what this means, and now, you also know how to manage it. You are armed with resources, apps, and recipes to help you along this lifelong journey. Food is not your enemy; it's your friend.

Cook your way to health and vitality with these recipes and tips. Good things are made to share, so please help a friend find out about this way of life. Call them over for a meal, talk about diabetes, and let's help create awareness as we feast on every delectable spoonful of diabetic cooking made easy.

Appendix 1: Measurement Conversion Chart

VOLUME EQUIVALENTS(DRY)

US STANDARD	METRIC (APPROXIMATE)
1/8 teaspoon	0.5 mL
1/4 teaspoon	1 mL
1/2 teaspoon	2 mL
3/4 teaspoon	4 mL
1 teaspoon	5 mL
1 tablespoon	15 mL
1/4 cup	59 mL
1/2 cup	118 mL
3/4 cup	177 mL
1 cup	235 mL
2 cups	475 mL
3 cups	700 mL
4 cups	1 L

VOLUME EQUIVALENTS(LIQUID)

US STANDARD	US STANDARD (OUNCES)	METRIC (APPROXIMATE)
2 tablespoons	1 fl.oz.	30 mL
1/4 cup	2 fl.oz.	60 mL
1/2 cup	4 fl.oz.	120 mL
1 cup	8 fl.oz.	240 mL
1 1/2 cup	12 fl.oz.	355 mL
2 cups or 1 pint	16 fl.oz.	475 mL
4 cups or 1 quart	32 fl.oz.	1 L
1 gallon	128 fl.oz.	4 L

TEMPERATURES EQUIVALENTS

FAHRENHEIT(F)	CELSIUS(C) (APPROXIMATE)
225 °F	107 °C
250 °F	120 °C
275 °F	135 °C
300 °F	150 °C
325 °F	160 °C
350 °F	180 °C
375 °F	190 °C
400 °F	205 °C
425 °F	220 °C
450 °F	235 °C
475 °F	245 °C
500 °F	260 °C

WEIGHT EQUIVALENTS

US STANDARD	METRIC (APPROXIMATE)
1 ounce	28 g
2 ounces	57 g
5 ounces	142 g
10 ounces	284 g
15 ounces	425 g
16 ounces (1 pound)	455 g

Appendix 2: The Dirty Dozen and Clean Fifteen

The Environmental Working Group (EWG) is a nonprofit, nonpartisan organization dedicated to protecting human health and the environment Its mission is to empower people to live healthier lives in a healthier environment. This organization publishes an annual list of the twelve kinds of produce, in sequence, that have the highest amount of pesticide residue-the Dirty Dozen-as well as a list of the fifteen kinds ofproduce that have the least amount of pesticide residue-the Clean Fifteen.

THE DIRTY DOZEN	THE CLEAN FIFTEEN
• The 2016 Dirty Dozen includes the following produce. These are considered among the year's most important produce to buy organic:	• The least critical to buy organically are the Clean Fifteen list. The following are on the 2016 list:

THE DIRTY DOZEN

Strawberries	Spinach
Apples	Tomatoes
Nectarines	Bell peppers
Peaches	Cherry tomatoes
Celery	Cucumbers
Grapes	Kale/collard greens
Cherries	Hot peppers

THE CLEAN FIFTEEN

Avocados	Papayas
Corn	Kiw
Pineapples	Eggplant
Cabbage	Honeydew
Sweet peas	Grapefruit
Onions	Cantaloupe
Asparagus	Cauliflower
Mangos	

• *The Dirty Dozen list contains two additional itemskale/collard greens and hot peppers-because they tend to contain trace levels of highly hazardous pesticides.*

• *Some of the sweet corn sold in the United States are made from genetically engineered (GE) seedstock. Buy organic varieties of these crops to avoid GE produce.*

Appendix 3: 4-Week Meal Plan

Week 1	Breakfast	Lunch	Dinner	Snack
1	Simple Grain-Free Biscuits	Eggplant-Zucchini Parmesan	Dandelion and Beet Greens with Black Beans	Cauliflower Mash
2	Banana Crêpe Cakes	Chipotle Chili Pork	Salmon Milano	Parmesan Crisps
3	Quick Breakfast Yogurt Sundae	Wilted Dandelion Greens with Sweet Onion	Grilled Shrimp Skewers	Caprese Skewers
4	Berry Bark	Cilantro Lime Shrimp	Chili Relleno Casserole	Aromatic Toasted Pumpkin Seeds
5	Easy Turkey Breakfast Patties	Wilted Dandelion Greens with Sweet Onion	Sautéed Zucchini and Tomatoes	Easy Low-Carb Biscuits
6	Tropical Yogurt Kiwi Bowl	Pulled Pork Sandwiches with Apricot Jelly	Grilled Tuna Steaks	Hot Chicken Stuffed Celery Stalks
7	Brussels Sprout with Fried Eggs	Butter-Lemon Grilled Cod on Asparagus	Seared Scallops with Orange Sauce	Bacon-Wrapped Shrimps

Week 2	Breakfast	Lunch	Dinner	Snack
1	Cauliflower Hash	Chipotle Chili Pork	Roasted Pork Loin with Carrots	Deviled Eggs
2	Coconut Porridge	Asparagus and Scallop Skillet with Lemony	Cheesy Mushroom and Pesto Flatbreads	Apple Pita Pockets
3	Scrambled Egg Whites with Bell Pepper	Zucchini and Pinto Bean Casserole	Cherry-Glazed Lamb Chops	Almond Cheesecake Bites
4	Ham and Jicama Hash	Lemon Parsley White Fish Fillets	Cod Fillet with Quinoa and Asparagus	Asian Chicken Wings
5	Feta Brussels Sprouts and Scrambled Eggs	Lemon Wax Beans	Easy Lime Lamb Cutlets	Hot Chicken Stuffed Celery Stalks
6	Berry Bark	Cajun Catfish	Fresh Rosemary Trout	Parmesan Crisps
7	Ham and Cheese Breakfast Biscuits	Lamb and Mushroom CheeseBurgers	Green Salmon Florentine	Easy Low-Carb Biscuits

Week 3	Breakfast	Lunch	Dinner	Snack
1	Peanut Butter and Berry Oatmeal	Parmesan Golden Pork Chops	Pork Loin, Carrot, and Gold Tomato Roast	Cauliflower Mash
2	Banana Crêpe Cakes	Eggplant-Zucchini Parmesan	Grilled Lamb Racks	Asian Chicken Wings
3	Cottage Pancakes	Pulled Pork Sandwiches with Apricot Jelly	Marinated Grilled Salmon with Lemongrass	Bacon-Wrapped Shrimps
4	Cranberry Grits	Wilted Dandelion Greens with Sweet Onion	Bacon and Cauliflower Casserole	Aromatic Toasted Pumpkin Seeds
5	Easy and Creamy Grits	Butter Cod with Asparagus	Fried Rice with Snap Peas	Caprese Skewers
6	Simple Cottage Cheese Pancakes	Cilantro Lime Shrimp	Mustard Pork Chops	Kale Chips
7	Tropical Yogurt Kiwi Bowl	Cajun Catfish	Chili Relleno Casserole	Asian Chicken Wings

Week 4	Breakfast	Lunch	Dinner	Snack
1	Feta Brussels Sprouts and Scrambled Eggs	Spaghetti Squash and Chickpea Bolognese	Seared Scallops with Orange Sauce	Almond Cheesecake Bites
2	Coconut Porridge	Creamy Cod Fillet with Quinoa and Asparagus	Cod Fillet with Quinoa and Asparagus	Deviled Eggs
3	Peanut Butter and Berry Oatmeal	Wilted Dandelion Greens with Sweet Onion	Easy Lime Lamb Cutlets	Bacon-Wrapped Shrimps
4	Ham and Jicama Hash	Grilled Portobello and Zucchini Burger	Grilled Tuna Steaks.	Apple Pita Pockets
5	Goat Cheese and Avocado Toast	Butter-Lemon Grilled Cod on Asparagus	Green Salmon Florentine	Kale Chips
6	Ham and Cheese Breakfast Biscuits	Zucchini and Pinto Bean Casserole	Pork Loin, Carrot, and Gold Tomato Roast	Caprese Skewers
7	Scrambled Egg Whites with Bell Pepper	Asparagus with Scallops	Grilled Lamb Racks	Cauliflower Mash

Appendix 4: Recipe Index

CPSIA information can be obtained
at www.ICGtesting.com
Printed in the USA
LVHW060826070421
683682LV00003B/105

9 781637 330111